Case Studies on the
BUSINESS OF NUTRACEUTICALS, FUNCTIONAL AND SUPER FOODS

WOODHEAD PUBLISHING SERIES IN CONSUMER SCIENCE AND STRATEGIC MARKETING

Case Studies on the BUSINESS OF NUTRACEUTICALS, FUNCTIONAL AND SUPER FOODS

Edited by

CRISTINA SANTINI
University San Raffaele Rome, Italy

STEFANIA SUPINO
University San Raffaele Rome, Italy

LUCIA BAILETTI
Sensory Consumer & Neuromarketing, Intertek Italia

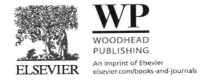

ELSEVIER

WP
WOODHEAD
PUBLISHING
An imprint of Elsevier
elsevier.com/books-and-journals

Woodhead Publishing
Woodhead Publishing is an imprint of Elsevier
50 Hampshire Street, 5th Floor, Cambridge, MA 02139, United States
The Boulevard, Langford Lane, Kidlington, OX5 1GB, United Kingdom

Notices
Knowledge and best practice in this field are constantly changing. As new research and experience broaden our understanding, changes in research methods, professional practices, or medical treatment may become necessary.

Practitioners and researchers must always rely on their own experience and knowledge in evaluating and using any information, methods, compounds, or experiments described herein. In using such information or methods they should be mindful of their own safety and the safety of others, including parties for whom they have a professional responsibility.

To the fullest extent of the law, neither the Publisher nor the authors, contributors, or editors, assume any liability for any injury and/or damage to persons or property as a matter of products liability, negligence or otherwise, or from any use or operation of any methods, products, instructions, or ideas contained in the material herein.

ISBN: 978-0-12-821408-4

For Information on all Woodhead Publishing publications visit our website at https://www.elsevier.com/books-and-journals

Publisher: Nikki P. Levy
Acquisitions Editor: Megan R. Ball
Editorial Project Manager: Lindsay C. Lawrence
Production Project Manager: Surya Narayanan Jayachandran
Cover Designer: Mark Rogers

Working together
to grow libraries in
developing countries
www.elsevier.com • www.bookaid.org

Typeset by Aptara, New Delhi, India

Contents

SECTION 2 Strategy

Contributors

Luciana Almeida
ESPM, Sao Paulo, Brazil

Lucia Bailetti
Sensory Consumer & Neuromarketing, Intertek Italia

Sergio Barile
Sapienza University, Rome, Italy

Joe Bogue
Department of Food Business and Development, Cork University Business School, University College Cork, Ireland

Lisa Callagher
University of Auckland, New Zealand

Maurizio Canavari
Department of Agricultural and Food Sciences, Alma Mater Studiorum-University of Bologna, Bologna, Italy

Giovani Caprioli
School of Pharmacy, Universiy of Camerino, Camerino, Italy

Alessandra Castellini
Department of Agricultural and Food Sciences, Alma Mater Studiorum-University of Bologna, Bologna, Italy

Manoel Messias Cavalcante
ESPM, Sao Paulo, Brazil

Alessio Cavicchi
Department of Agriculture, Food and Environment, University of Pisa, Pisa, Italy

Ziad Elsahn
Northumbria University, Newcastle Business School, United Kingdom

Eduardo de Rezende Francisco
FGV EAESP, Sao Paulo, Brazil

Stefan Korber
University of Auckland, New Zealand

Filippo Maggi
School of Pharmacy, Universiy of Camerino, Camerino, Italy

Ornella Malandrino
DISA-MIS, University of Salerno, Fisciano, SA, Italy

Astride Franks Kamgang Nzekoue
School of Pharmacy, Universiy of Camerino, Camerino, Italy

Riccardo Petrelli
School of Pharmacy, Universiy of Camerino, Camerino, Italy

Francesco Polese
DISA-MIS, University of Salerno, Fisciano, SA, Italy

Lana Repar
Department of Food Business and Development, Cork University Business School, University College Cork, Ireland

Gianni Sagratini
School of Pharmacy, Universiy of Camerino, Camerino, Italy

Cristina Santini
University San Raffaele Rome, Italy

Frank Siedlok
Heriot-Watt University, Edinburgh, United Kingdom

Stefania Supino
University San Raffaele Rome, Italy

Mario Testa
DISA-MIS, University of Salerno, Fisciano, SA, Italy

Sauro Vittori
School of Pharmacy, Universiy of Camerino, Camerino, Italy

Vilma Xhakollari
Department of Agricultural and Food Sciences, Alma Mater Studiorum-University of Bologna, Bologna, Italy

Introduction

The nutraceutical and superfood industries have boomed.

This book wants to highlight the challenges and opportunities of the nutraceutical business. The chapter entitled "The Market" provides an overview of market trends. It explores the forces and the drivers that have made this business one of the most attractive and profitable businesses of the last decade. The blurring of industries (food, pharma, and cosmetics) has created new market opportunities for business players. This dynamic industry has seen further development with the pandemic event since consumers' attention to healthy issues has increased. The intensification of competition and highly innovative products launched on the market requires particular attention to customers' needs. It emerges how pivotal it is to explore consumers' preferences and orientations. The chapter entitled "A Short Review of Willingness to Pay for Novel Foods" illustrates the state of the art of background research on consumers' willingness to pay for novel foods. It introduces a problem that often emerges in the book: the relationship between consumers and novel foods and consequently neophobia in food products. The analysis of the main findings of willingness to pay helps understand how consumers shape their preferences and manage information when marketing novel foods. The role that information covers in developing this industry emerges in several chapters in the book. For example, it is highly relevant for companies trying to strategically use traditional food benefits (as we see in the chapter "Typical Plant-based Food from a Nutraceutical Perspective: The Case of the Marche Region"). Another example is in the chapter that explores the case study of an Italian company, the Severino Becagli (see the chapter "Organic and Made in Tuscany Spirulina: The Story of Severino Becagli"). This company is trying to combine the country of origin with organic certification and nutraceutical benefits in its marketing strategy.

New product development (NPD) is a key issue in this industry.

This book (see the chapters entitled "Market-oriented Methodologies that Integrate the Consumer into the Functional Foods New Product Development Process: Part 1 and Part 2") remarks on the importance of market orientation for developing new functional foods.

Implementing methodologies that can generate the consumer's voice can be highly fruitful for companies. Companies should understand how to develop information from consumers. What is the role of research in this scenario? How can research help in the generation of information? The chapters mentioned above describe the methodologies that can be employed for assisting companies in NPD. The chapter describes what method best fits the NPD stage and the questions each tool addresses.

The chapter's strategic relevance of a market-oriented approach to developing functional foods emerges. The growing demand for functional foods is determined by motivated consumers who seek healthy lifestyles. It is essential to understand what consumers want: developing products following the idea that given the general interest, new products will encounter a consensus in the market, which can be hazardous.

The importance of consumer orientation also emerges from the chapter entitled "Competitive Advantage Through Multidisciplinary Innovation in Nutraceuticals: From Concept Optimization to Context Transformation," illustrating how a multidisciplinary approach could be beneficial. Being consumer-oriented implies an accurate analysis of consumer behavior and preferences and reshaping the company's entire management by introducing a new and broader perspective. The chapter highlights that a multidisciplinary approach to innovation could work to support with evidence health claims as required by legislative frameworks. Multidisciplinarity and open innovation require an accurate reflection on the implications that they could have for companies' management. As it emerges from the chapter, a multidisciplinary approach is crucial for optimizing technical aspects, especially in NPD or nutraceutical innovation.

The signs of progress in the nutraceutical industry have opened a debate about food security and safety. From the book, we learn about nutraceuticals and superfoods' role in ensuring access to nutrients among various populations. This is a promising and exciting research field that will have further development in the future.

Therefore, the book explores another aspect: the ability to revitalize typical mature products by using nutraceutical components as leverages. The two chapters, "The LBG Case Study" and "Typical Plant-based Food from a Nutraceutical Perspective: The Case of the Marche Region," show how to employ consumer science for rejuvenating mature products.

As we have seen from this introduction, the business of nutraceuticals and superfoods is extraordinarily dynamic and competitive. Nevertheless, competitive advantage is of primary importance in the business: the business attracts competitors, and producers need to maintain excellent market orientation. In this scenario, adopting a multidisciplinary perspective on the business is mandative: the collaboration between strategic marketing and consumer science appears to be highly fruitful.

SECTION 1

The scenario

CHAPTER 1

The Nutraceutical Industry: trends and dynamics

Cristina Santini[a], Stefania Supino[a], Lucia Bailetti[b]
[a]University San Raffaele Rome, Italy
[b]Sensory Consumer & Neuromarketing, Intertek Italia

1.1 Introduction

The business of nutraceuticals, which includes a broad range of products, such as dietary supplements, functional beverages and foods or superfoods, is growing. The growing demand for nutraceuticals will be a key driving factor for the global market. It will mainly involve the food and pharmaceutical industries; the nutraceutical sector, indeed, has arisen at the boundaries of these industries since the early 1990s.

The relationship between food and health is the cornerstone of the nutraceutical sector.

Drivers of the growth of the global nutraceutical market are multifactorial. However, they can be summarised by four main themes: the ageing of the population; increasing healthcare costs; increasing distribution channels; consumer lifestyle, and consumer awareness. Consumers have progressively adopted behaviours to prevent diseases and have become intensely aware of the importance of adopting healthy food consumption habits. Their attention is focused on how foods can contribute to health, wellness, and the positive impact some types of food could have in preventing healthy diseases. Nutraceuticals are also beneficial in inappropriate lifestyles, nutritional intake, and specific situations, such as intense sports practice, pregnancy, or postmenopause.

This chapter will provide an overview of the business of nutraceuticals and functional foods. Following emerging insights from the literature, we will outline the evolutionary paths of the industry, and we will provide an overview of the competitive dynamics of the business.

Case Studies on the Business of Nutraceuticals, Functional and Super Foods
DOI: https://doi.org/10.1016/B978-0-12-821408-4.00006-7

1.2 Definitions

In the literature, many works define nutraceuticals, functional foods, and superfoods.

Sometimes (see among the others Hardy, 2000), the terms are employed as synonymous or are incorrectly used[a]. Despite rising public interest in nutraceuticals, the lack of universally accepted definitions remains a challenge.

There is an agreement (Kalra, 2003) about the recognition who has firstly introduced the term "nutraceutical": De Felice in the eighties was the first to refer to nutraceuticals as "a food (or part of a food) that provides medical or health benefits, including the prevention and/or treatment of a disease".

In the absence of an internationally shared definition of nutraceuticals (Aronson, 2017), it is now commonly used to refer to the "nutritional products that provide health and medical benefits, including the prevention and treatment of disease", according to the European Nutraceutical Association (2016). In other words, as Santini and Novellino (2017) underline, nutraceuticals position themselves beyond the diet and before the drug.

Some of these products can be found in nature and extracted, and, following clinical evidence, they can be finally sold under a pharmaceutical form. The strong connection with food products and their natural origins have created contact points between the food and the pharmaceutical industries. Consequently, a system of relationships and contaminations has emerged, and it has redefined the innovative orientation of the firms competing in the industry.

Following the needs emerging from longer life expectancy, food functionalities and its physiological functions attract consumers. In addition, these compounds are characterized by negligible side effects compared to traditional pharmacological therapies, so consumers lean towards their use for health promotion. One of the pioneer countries for functional food production was Japan (Menrad, 2003): Japan introduced in the 1980s functional foods in the market by defining them "any food or ingredient

---

[a]Hardy (2000) in particular refer to the incorrect employment of terms such as "Functional foods", "nutraceuticals", "pharmaconutrients", and "dietary integrators" and more specifically: "Functional foods", "nutraceuticals", "pharmaconutrients", and "dietary integrators" are all terms used incorrectly and indiscriminately for nutrients or nutrient-enriched foods that can prevent or treat diseases" (p. 69).

that has a positive impact on an individual's health, physical performance, or state of mind, in addition to its nutritive value" (p. 687, Hardy, 2000).

The International Food Information Council (IFIC) provides a useful definition of functional food that highlights the benefit associated with nutrition: functional foods are foods or dietary components that may benefit health beyond basic nutrition. Other provided definitions underline the aspect of physiological benefits associated with functional foods: the International Life Science Institute of North America defines functional foods as "foods that by virtue of physiologically active food components provide health benefits beyond basic nutrition".

The *Nutrition Business Journal* defines functional foods as "food fortified with added or concentrated ingredients to functional levels, which improves health or performance".

As we can see, the concept of benefit is at the base of all the previously provided definitions: consumers, when they intake specific nutrients or foods, receive a health benefit. The aspect of convenience when assuming nutraceuticals or functional food emerges from the definition that El Sohaimy (2012) provides: "Functional foods, on the other hand, are products that are consumed as foods and not in dosage form (p. 692)". This last underlined aspect is extremely helpful because it suggests that the consumers cannot take the components available in functional foods by using any other way than feeding.

Therefore, following what emerges from the literature, we can distinguish other subcategories that include functional foods in the nutraceuticals category.

There are many taxonomies of nutraceuticals, and they vary according to the approach.

According to Gupta et al. (2010), nutraceuticals can be classified according to chemical constituents—and we find three main categories, nutrients, herbal and dietary supplements—or to tradition—so they can be traditional or nontraditional. The traditional ones are, for example, nutrients, herbals, phytochemicals, probiotic microorganisms, nutraceutical enzymes, and the nontraditional or artificial nutraceuticals are, for example, fortified and recombinant nutraceuticals (Alamgir, 2017).

1.3 Market

Nutraceuticals represent a profitable and growing market: although it is difficult to find some precise information about the value of the market at a global level, we know, for sure, that it is growing and attracts many competitors.

In 2020, the global market size for nutraceuticals products was valued 412.7 billion US dollars. Projections for the period 2020–25 show a CAGR of 8.3% [b]. It is challenging to find harmonized data that analyse the dimensions of the industry: data differ by source, and it is hard to find free information about this industry. According to KPMG, the United States represents the leading market for nutraceuticals, followed by Japan and Europe. The trends that emerge from the analysis of the European dietary supplement market (fortune business insights) highlight a considerable value projected to reach 33.80 Bn USD by 2027 with a CAGR of 9.3% in the period 2019–27[c].

The European market sees the UK as major players (with an expected CAGR in the period 2020–27 of 9.69%), Germany, Italy, France, and Spain. Some countries, such as Greece, The Netherlands, Ireland, Denmark, Poland, Austria, or Belgium, are seeing a diffusion of supplements among consumers. As we can see, there is a positive trend for the consumption and diffusion of nutraceuticals, but it is clear, as Menrad (2003) underlines, this is a scattered market.

The market results from a blurring of different industries (Fig. 1.1), in particular pharmaceutical and nutrition. However, we are also assisting with the emerging role of the personal care industry. Many companies can simultaneously operate in the Cosmeceuticals, Nutraceuticals, and Nutricosmetics field[d].

Given the described scenario, it is clear that different motivations shape consumption and range from health concerns to nutritional issues.

The nutraceutical market includes different categories of products; the food segment has a leading role in the growth of the business in 2019 (BusinessWire). Consumers' attention towards health and nutritional issues has motivated the booming of product categories, such as snacks with

---

[b]The source of information is Grandview research (https://www.grandviewresearch.com/industry-analysis/nutraceuticals-market). Other companies (see https://www.globenewswire.com/news-release/2021/06/17/2249181/0/en/Nutraceuticals-Market-Size-Worth-Around-US-314-2-Bn-by-2030.html) provides different projection, with a CAGR of 7.2% In the period 2019–25 for a global value of 404.8 billion USD. It is hard to find commonly shared information about the global value and growth of the industry; in any case the trend is extremely positive.

[c]For more information : https://www.fortunebusinessinsights.com/industry-reports/europe-dietary-supplements-market-101918.

[d]An example is the French company Biocyte (https://www.biocyte.com).

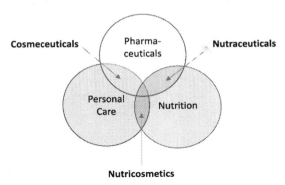

Fig. 1.1 *The blurring of industries.*

functional ingredients. According to BusinessWire, conventional stores will play a leading role in the distribution of nutraceuticals: according to AC Nielsen, retailers are becoming health care providers in the United States, given the space they dedicate on their shelves to nutraceuticals and functional food products. Supplements represent a growing opportunity for retailers (https://www.supermarketnews.com/health-wellness/supplements-big-growth-opportunities-grocery-retailers) and by improving the availability of these categories of products in their store, retailers have facilitated consumers accessibility to nutraceuticals.

The nutraceutical industry is largely consumer-driven and will continue to grow because it fits the current lifestyle of developing and developed countries (Chopra et al., 2022). Given the above-described scenario, we can say that the business of nutraceuticals is dynamic, and its growth depends on the characteristics that each category of products has on a geographical base. In particular, the diffusion of some specific diseases in some populations is related to diffused food consumption habits and nutritional and health concerns. Consequently, the local population's socio-demographic characteristics shape demand for nutraceuticals. Due to differences in local consumers' profiles and needs, some products might reach a wide diffusion in some geographical regions instead of others.

Moreover, consumer awareness has mainly driven the growth of the nutraceutical market since the beginning of the COVID-19 pandemic. The 2019 coronavirus disease (COVID-19, caused by SARS-CoV-2) is an easily transmissible disease that was identified in December 2019 and acknowledged as a pandemic by WHO in March 2020. The Covid-19 pandemic led to lockdowns in large parts of the world to contain or reduce the rate of viral transmission, radically transforming several people's lifestyles and daily habits, overall dietary profiles, and consumer behaviour patterns. Due to many countries experiencing successive waves of infection, the health crisis has represented an essential accelerator towards a reconfiguration of nutraceuticals market spaces, giving significant impulse to existing consumer phenomena and behaviours (Galanakis, 2020). An unprecedented rise in consumer sales of supplementary nutrients, nutraceutical products, and functional foods that were considered effective against the virus emerged. For example, in the United States, sales of supplements and nutraceuticals grew by 51.2% at the start of the pandemic in March 2020 compared to 2019 and remained high as evident by the 16.7% growth in July 2020. In Europe, China, and India, similar trends emerged. In this scenario, an intense debate on the efficacy and safety of nutraceuticals for the prevention and/or treatment of COVID-19 is ongoing. Sales of nutraceuticals were expected to remain high in the first half of 2021, albeit at a much lower level than the sales achieved at the beginning of the pandemic (Chopra et al., 2022).

1.4 Industry, competitive dynamics, and innovation

The industry system includes different types of stakeholders.

Producing companies that converge from other businesses or are born to play in the business must design a product portfolio marketed through direct or indirect sale channels to the final consumer. Competitive dynamics characterise the business ecosystem. Companies have to manage their product portfolio that could include a brand new product or focus on expanding the product portfolio. Companies could also go for a consolidation of the offer and the presence on the markets. This was, in general, the dynamics that operating companies must face and Fig. 1.2 represents the starting point for further reflections on the industry's competitive dynamics.

1.4.1 Regulatory framework

The characteristics of the business ecosystem shape firms' competitiveness. As in any other industry, in the nutraceutical business, suppliers and manufacturers play a crucial role in creating competitive advantage; thus, this industry is characterised by a critical situation for what concerns regulatory framework. There is a lack of a regulatory framework among countries.

Regulation changes according to the considered country: for example, in the United States, the Food and Drug Administration employs a specific set of regulations for nutraceuticals that cover many aspects of production

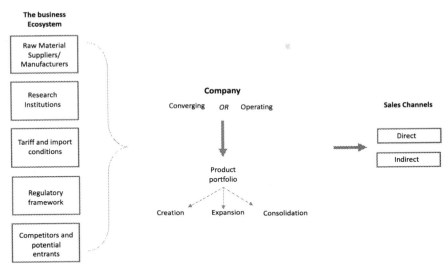

Fig. 1.2 *The industry system.*

included final product safety[c]. In the European Union, the approach to nutraceuticals is closer to the adopted approach for food; instead, Canada is nearer to drugs. In the Asia–Pacific region, Japan was among the first countries to face the issue of regulating food supplements and foodstuff by their regulatory authority, the Foods for Specified Health Use (FOSHU).

[c]The article published on the news-medical.net (https://www.news-medical.net/health/Nutraceutical-Regulation.aspx) illustrates the process: "In the United States, the Food and Drug Administration (FDA) regulates nutraceuticals under a different set of regulations as compared to those that cover "conventional" food and drug products. According to the Dietary Supplement Health and Education Act from 1994 (DSHEA), it is the manufacturer's responsibility to ensure that a nutraceutical is safe before it is marketed. The FDA is authorized to take action against any unsafe product after it reaches the market. Manufacturers have to make sure that the information on the product label is truthful and not misleading; however, they are not obliged to register their products with the FDA nor get FDA approval before producing or selling nutraceuticals. In the European Union (EU), food legislation is largely under the umbrella of the European Food and Safety Authority (EFSA). This legislation focuses on "food supplements", which are defined as concentrated sources of nutrients like proteins, minerals, and vitamins, as well as other substances that offer a beneficial nutritional effect. The main EU legislation related to food supplements is Directive 2002/46/EC. New products from Europe are presumed to have passed stringent European development and quality requirements. As a result, European nutraceutical companies, which are generally considered leaders in innovation, enjoy the public perception that they are producing the highest quality products. In Canada and Australia, nutraceuticals are regulated more closely as a drug than food category".

Many other countries, such as Australia or China, regulate nutraceuticals simply as a food category. Other countries do not have specific regulations (Chopra et al., 2022). This scenario feeds uncertainty in the business and could create additional costs. There is a case that underlines the relationship between regulatory framework and costs. In 2012, the European Food Safety Authority revised labelling requirements for probiotics to improve the effectiveness of health claims information. This has meant for probiotic producers to be compelled to provide a considerable amount of scientific evidence to support health claims, which means, in other words, investing in testing and research.

Some countries are working for improving the regulatory system to make information more clear and help companies to reduce costs.[f] As it emerges from the published report of the UK government, the creation of "a new regulatory framework for the fast-growing category of novel health-enhancing foods and supplements to promote investment in the UK as a leader in the nutraceutical sector". The UK has recognised that the traditional silos of regulatory classifications are challenged by "the pace of bioscience and technological convergence of biological and digital platforms" (p. 109). Therefore, a revision of the regulatory process for nutraceuticals could represent leverage for improving the competitive advantage of a country.

1.4.2 Industry convergence and new entrants

Competitive dynamics in this industry are particularly complex.

As mentioned above, there is a blurring of industry boundaries occurring in the nutraceutical sector.

In one of its published reports, Price Water House underlines that nutraceutical—as well as cosmeceutical and nutracosmetical—is born as an innovative and transversal segment to other industries (Pharmaceutical, Nutrition, and Personal Care). Innovativeness is, therefore, one of the characteristics of this industry, together with convergence.

The phenomenon of industry convergence in the nutraceutical business is not new to the literature. In particular, the work by Bröring et al. (2006) highlights that in the nutraceutical industry, technology, and demand structure converge: on one side, producers that operate in the food and pharmaceutical industries develop new functional or nutraceutical products; on the

---

[f]https://assets.publishing.service.gov.uk/government/uploads/system/uploads/attachment_data/file/994125/FINAL_TIGRR_REPORT__1_.pdf.

other consumers seek for single products that provide multiple answers to a wide range of needs (Hilton, 2017) talks about convergence in categories, channels, technologies, and consumers.

In this scenario, new entrants can gain a profitable market share.

Some corporations are financing start-ups for entering this industry: Nestlè, for example, has created a venture capital fund for investing in early stage nutraceutical businesses[g] and in 2019 the corporation has funded an R&D acceleration in Lausanne (Switzerland) to work in collaboration with some academic institution such as the Swiss Federal Institute of Technology in Lausanne (EPFL) and Zurich (ETHZ) or the Swiss Hospitality Management School in Lausanne.

However, the competitive landscape is characterized by the presence of key international players. Companies have implemented mergers & acquisitions and new product launches as key strategies to compete in the market. Mergers & acquisitions enabled the companies to expand their product's array and improve product quality, meeting the changing consumer trends across the industry (www.grandviewresearch.com/industry-analysis/nutraceuticals-market).

1.4.3 New products

Companies operating in this field must pay particular attention to needs that emerge from the market and trends in demand.

To provide a clear example, we can underline that operators in the industry are assisting to a progressive redefinition of health priorities (https://www.nutraceuticalsworld.com/issues/2019-09/view_features/resetting-nutraceutical-industry-priorities/): mental and emotional health is becoming a primary need for consumers who are adopting a holistic approach to health and nutrition. This segment in 2019 grew up to gain a share of 40% in the US adult population: it is clear that industry players are adapting their offer. Millennials and GenZ also need to manage stress and anxiety. In general, the issue of mental wellbeing is reshaping nutraceuticals.

The openness to innovation that characterises the industry creates a breeding ground for the proliferation of new products to be launched on the market.

In the above-described scenario, companies should manage some risks. The first risk concerns the length of the product life cycle: where

---

[g]For more information: https://www.inventages.com/about-us/.

the degree of innovation is exceptionally high, products, in general, have shorter life cycles.

About the threat of substitute products, we can say that the cost of nutraceuticals can be higher than the one of active pharmaceuticals ingredients due to the high content of technology in the extracting process (https://www.globenewswire.com/news-release/2021/06/08/2243610/0/en/Global-Nutraceutical-Ingredients-Market-Growing-Steadily-Amid-the-Ongoing-Pandemic-Projected-to-Reach-USD-208-2-Billion-by-2027.html).

Consequently, in the long run, some changes in the competitive asset of the industry can happen. It can stimulate a process of product substitution. In general, the threat of substitute products could seriously reduce the industry's profitability.

The industry is particularly dynamic, and new product categories emerge: to support this evidence, there is an extensive number of classifications of nutraceuticals. Market demand stimulates the creation of new products, as evidenced by the literature (see among the others, Hilton, 2017).

Today professionals must deal with categories such as "better for you" (food that contains less or none of an ingredient, such as sodium, fat, or sugar) or "added functionality" (we refer to food with added fibre, calcium, vitamins, or antioxidant), terms that today are currently employed, but that a few years ago were new to producers. In other words, while initially nutraceuticals were classified according to some general principles (type or application), today, the emerging of market needs has contributed to the development of some different ways to market products to make them more accessible and understandable. The consumption of nutraceuticals can be daily or finalised for a specific purpose; this has got some implications on packaging or format to ease consumption and reduce its complexity when consumption is by day.

Another important trend emerging from the market is embracing sustainability as a business imperative, adopting models that create shared value and drive systemic changes towards green and circular economy goals. The latter requires the rethinking of production, consumption, and waste management systems, embracing reliable tools that can support organisations in decision-making processes, complementing economic, environmental, and social dimensions.

The literature analysed sustainability approaches and business challenges related to the nutraceutical industry. Galanakis (2013) investigates emerging technologies for producing nutraceuticals from agricultural by-products.

Mirabella et al. (2014) proposed the development of innovative nutritional by-products from food waste using the circular economy approach. Mutalipassi et al. (2021) focused on the possible valorisation of seafood by-products as a source of biomolecules, valid for the sustainable production of high-value nutraceutical compounds. Chang et al. (2015) demonstrated the use of carbon footprint to improve the environmental performance of the nutraceutical industry. Varela-Candamio et al. (2018) proposed a business conceptual framework that manages the generation-production-consumption of nutraceuticals, involving rural women and promoting social targets. Chaurasia et al. (2021) focused on nutraceutical managerial research within the context of United Nations Sustainable Development Goals-2030. This study highlights that nutraceuticals were initially developed to improve nutritional programs among undernourished poor populations of low-income countries. Today, industrialised nations represent the leading producers and consumers of nutraceutical products. Consumers in developing countries command a mere 2%–3% share of the global market.

The nutraceutical industry shows consistent progress towards sustainability: the speciality chemicals industry supply valued ingredients obtained from biological resources previously discarded as waste. Companies in the business are also adopting eco-friendly packaging options to offer ecological benefits in addition to standard product benefits (Pagliaro, 2020).

Evidence of this ongoing change ranging from the extraction of fish oil from fish and crustacean processing leftovers, rather than contributing to overfishing of several marine species (Ciriminna et al., 2017), to obtaining olive polyphenols from olive mill wastewater, closing the production cycle and obtaining polyphenol extracts with an exceptionally high load (Delisi et al., 2018).

1.5 Determinants of growth

As we have seen, it is challenging to define the boundaries of nutraceuticals, functional, and superfoods. Therefore, we will examine some of the issues that motivate the growth of this industry and explain the presence of variation in product demand among different segments of the population or geographical areas.

1.5.1 The mix with cultural and societal issues

There are many reasons behind the growing popularity and interest in Nutraceuticals, functional, and superfoods. One of the issues at the base of the positive market trends of these products is the perfect integration of some product features with consumers cultural issues.

Some countries have developed traditional medical systems and have stressed the importance of food as a critical asset to gain and maintain health. For example, the presence of Ayurveda principles in the cultural roots of the population in the Indian Subcontinent has represented, over the centuries, a breeding ground for developing attention for nutraceutical and functional components of food. As mentioned by Payyappallimana and Venkatasubramanian (2016), one of the precepts of Ayurveda is the classification of food according to both organoleptic properties and the related impact of individual's psychological constitution. There is an open debate on the relationship between traditional and modern medicines (see, e.g., the work by Pandey et al., 2013). We should underline that a cultural orientation towards the importance of nutrients and food has nurtured the interest in nutraceuticals and functional foods. This interest has represented the basis for reinforcing a growing market. India represents a key player in this industry. We can make similar considerations for the role of traditional medicine in China; we also have previously cited Japan, where the term functional food was first coined. In Japan, there is a diffused cultural attention towards the link between food and health. According to some authors (Ohama et al., 2006), this trend is so relevant that in Japan, people employ the generic term "health food" to describe "functional food".

Also, in other cultures, inspired by religious motives, people seek nutraceuticals or functional food to maintain healthy status, following what their credo suggests them. According to Hasnah Hassan (2011), religious principles foster the adoption of healthy food consumption and the awareness towards functional and nutraceutical foods in Malaysian Muslims.

Another interesting aspect to consider is the widespread diffusion of knowledge about positive interactions between nutrients or types of foods, which can affect people's health. The existence of cultural issues that link territories with cultivars and agricultural products that belong to the heritage of some rural communities has reinforced the linkage between people and food products, especially when it is proven that they can provide benefits for health.

1.5.2 Changes in communication

In a report published by the IFIC, we can read: " How nutrition information is shared also seems to affect the degree to which the information is trusted" (https://foodinsight.org/wp-content/uploads/2017/05/2017-ExSum-FoodConfusion.pdf). There is a discrepancy between trusted and reliable information. There are many sources of information (professionals, family and friends, government and agencies, socials), and they do not have the same level of accuracy and reliability. The work by Annunziata and Vecchio (2011) highlights the role that different sources of information can have in shaping consumers' purchasing intention of functional foods.

Consumers need to assess the reliability of the source of information; secondly, consumers should adopt behaviours aligned to the provided advice. As the IFIC has underlined, in some cases, the people you trust do not promote nutrition habits coherent with the issues emerging from professionals and doctors.

The diffusion of media and social media has created a proliferation of information about health issues. On one side, many companies and operators in the nutraceutical and functional food business have realized that since people spend more time watching socials, the importance of socials in communication grows. On the other side, the interest in health issues among social media users has represented a way for many social media professionals to reach new contacts.

For the first category of people—professionals in nutrition and food—social media have represented a tool for getting in touch with consumers; for the second category—social media professionals—healthy issues have represented a means for gaining new contacts.

This has nourished further confusion: consumers should ask whom to trust and why. The critical question should be provided recommendations are based on trustable scientific information or not? Given the lack of a clear definition of the contents of labels for functional and nutraceutical foods (see among the others, Naylor et al., 2009), consumers have searched for information through different sources.

The continuous evolution of communication means and social media has reshaped the relationship between consumers and information. Professionals and educators have started to exploit and investigate the possibilities offered by the web and social media for diffusing information and nutritional programs: we can cite the case of Food Hero, described by Tobey Lauren and Manore Melinda (2014).

We have assisted to the growth of a collaborative intent in defining contents of news and info with the growth of social media, for example, we have seen the diffusion of collaborative journalism, where professional journalists collaborate with ordinary people that become reporters (Rutsaert et al., 2013). The example of collaborative journalism shows how information is created and the role of media in this process. We can see some similar aspects in nutraceuticals and functional foods: people that belong to various groups (professionals, consumers, influencers, doctors, industry, and so forth) contribute to creating information about single products. Consumers can gain information from different sources and then employ them to evaluate a product and purchase it. On one side, it could become highly complicated for consumers to understand what is reliable and trustable and what is not adequately supported by scientific evidence; on the other, the amount of information grew and its accessibility.

1.5.3 Preventive approach

Consumers' concerns about health stimulated a shift from a reactive to a preventive approach to healthcare. In this scenario, the COVID-19 pandemic has accelerated an already approach to healthy eating, focusing consumers' attention on prevention of health conditions, vitamins/minerals, immunity, and consideration for at-risk individuals. Most important, it has skyrocketed the "food as medicine" movement. Urban people are concerned about their health. While the COVID has renewed interest in rural areas, due to the massive emerging of smart working, people are getting more interested in evaluating the benefits of nutraceuticals and functional foods for preventing diseases. As we can see from the latest news and reports, the recent evolution of the global crisis due to COVID has intensified the orientation towards a preventive approach to food and nutrition in general. The current global health situation has stimulated a debate on problems like obesity or diabetes. There is a consensus about the linkage between obesity and severe COVID19 disease (see, e.g., Stefan et al., 2021). In many cases, the limitation of physical activity has nurtured a sedentary lifestyle.

In a report that examines the nutraceutical market, Price Water House Coopers underlines the role that COVID has had in developing the market for vitamins and supplements that were supposed to stimulate resistance to the virus (https://www.pwc.com/it/it/publications/assets/docs/Vitamins-Dietary-Supplements-Market-Overview.pdf).

The growing costs of the traditional healthcare system motivate the need to prevent rather than react (https://www.who.int/news/item/20-02-2019-countries-are-spending-more-on-health-but-people-are-still-paying-too-much-out-of-their-own-pockets). Some countries, such as the United States, are experiencing a rise in the incidence of healthcare costs on GDP.

Several scholars have underlined that policymakers should carefully evaluate the implications of functional and nutraceuticals foods for the local populations.

In a report published in 2008 by JRC, we can read: "Yet, whether promoting functional food is an efficient way of improving public health in the first place is the subject of a debate that is in need of more research: while the general research output on functional food in the EU is bigger than in the United States or Japan, the scope of the potential impact and cost-effectiveness of functional food are little researched topics so far. Therefore it may be pertinent to focus on these issues to substantiate the economic rationale of functional foods from a public health perspective and to allow both policy makers and consumers make informed decisions" (p. 8).

Consumers recognise the importance of functional foods and nutraceuticals for preventing diseases and adopting a healthy lifestyle: therefore, it is essential for policymakers to ensure adequate and clear access to information for consumers and to support and promote the industry.

1.6 Conclusions

The business of nutraceuticals is extremely attractive for professionals and scholars. Professionals see in nutraceuticals a profitable opportunity: the market can ensure good margins, and it shows a positive trend. Furthermore, new market niches can emerge, bringing a lower degree of competition and competitive advantage at the initial stages of the process.

We have outlined the motivations behind the growing demand for nutraceuticals that are highly heterogeneous and, in some cases, are strictly related to socio-demographical characteristics of the population. The interest shown by multinational corporations and global players for this industry has stimulated further changes in the industry that cover different aspects, from research and development to product distribution.

On the other hand, scholars have outlined various research insights that emerge from the industry. Research has explored the medical and biological aspects of the components of nutraceuticals and different elements of the business: from competitive dynamics and category convergence to the role that research and development can have in creating nutraceutical food products.

After having outlined the market characteristics and the emerging threats and opportunities, some interesting insights emerge. First of all, given the positive role that nutraceuticals can have in preventing diseases, policy-makers should promote an adequate education and information for the employment of nutraceuticals in dietary habits. The debate on the lack of a regulatory framework is another interesting aspect: a commonly shared set of regulations can protect industry players and help consumers achieve clear information.

Therefore, the role of research is pivotal in this industry: the growing interest shown by global companies on one side stimulates the emerging of new products, on the other could increase a divarium between those companies who have limited access to resources for R&D due to their small size and those with indigenous resources. Collaborative research systems could be particularly helpful in this scenario and could also help smaller players.

We know, for sure, that the preventive approach is reshaping the entire health system, and this fully motivates a holistic approach to health where nutraceuticals will play a leading role.

Nevertheless, the advances in nutraceutical-based preventive and proactive approaches require reliable clinical data substantiating their efficacy. In this direction, the increasing cooperation between the pharma and nutraceutical industries contributes to reshaping the nutraceutical industry. The rising interest of pharmaceutical companies encourages advances in the nutraceutical industry that is moving in the direction of pharmaceuticals to be clinically supported and achieve higher quality, safety, and stability standards, and, ultimately, provide solid data. Simultaneously, nutraceuticals allow pharmaceutical companies to expand their target audience to a broader base of health-conscious people.

References

Alamgir, A.N.M, 2017. Classification of drugs, nutraceuticals, functional food, and cosmeceuticals; proteins, peptides, and enzymes as drugsTherapeutic Use of Medicinal Plants and Their Extracts, *Volume* 1. Springer, Cham, pp. 125–175.

Annunziata, A., Vecchio, R., 2011. Functional foods development in the European market: a consumer perspective. J. Functional Foods 3 (3), 223–228.

Aronson, J.K., 2017. Defining 'nutraceuticals': neither nutritious nor pharmaceutical. British J. Clin. Pharmacol. 83 (1), 8–19.

Bröring, S., Martin Cloutier, L., Leker, J., 2006. The front end of innovation in an era of industry convergence: evidence from nutraceuticals and functional foods. R&D Manag. 36 (5), 487–498.

Chaurasia, S., Pati, R.K., Padhi, S.S., Jensen, J.M., Gavirneni, N., 2021. Achieving the United Nations sustainable development goals-2030 through the nutraceutical industry: a review of managerial research and the role of operations management. Decision Sci. 2021, 1–16. doi:10.1111/deci.12515

Chang, D.S., Yeh, L.T., Liu, W., 2015. Incorporating the carbon footprint to measure industry context and energy consumption effect on environmental performance of business operations. Clean Technologies Environ. Policy 17 (2), 359–371.

Chopra, A.S., Lordan, R., Horbańczuk, O.K., Atanasov, A.G., Chopra, I., Horbańczuk, J.O...., Arkells, N., 2022. The current use and evolving landscape of nutraceuticals. Pharmacol. Res. 175, 106001.

Ciriminna, R., Meneguzzo, F., Delisi, R., Pagliaro, M., 2017. Enhancing and improving the extraction of omega-3 from fish oil. Sustain. Chem. Pharmacy 5, 54–59.

Delisi, R., Ciriminna, R., Arvati, S., Meneguzzo, F., Pagliaro, M., 2018. Olive biophenol integral extraction at a two-phase olive mill. J. Clean. Prod. 174, 1487–1491.

El Sohaimy, S.A., 2012. Functional foods and nutraceuticals-modern approach to food science. World Appl. Sci. J. 20 (5), 691–708.

Galanakis, C.M., 2013. Emerging technologies for the production of nutraceuticals from agricultural by-products: a viewpoint of opportunities and challenges. Food Bioproducts Process. 91 (4), 575–579.

Galanakis, C.M., 2020. The food systems in the era of the coronavirus (COVID-19) pandemic crisis. Foods 9 (4), 523.

Gupta, S., Chauhan, D., Mehla, K., Sood, P., Nair, A., 2010. An overview of nutraceuticals: current scenario. J. Basic Clinical Pharm. 1 (2), 55.

Hardy, G., 2000. Nutraceuticals and functional foods: introduction and meaning. Nutrition 16 (7), 688–689.

Hasnah Hassan, S., 2011. Consumption of functional food model for Malay Muslims in Malaysia. J. Islamic Market. 2 (2), 104–124.

Hilton, J., 2017. Growth patterns and emerging opportunities in nutraceutical and functional food categories: market overview. In: Bagchi, D., Nair, S. (Eds.), Developing New Functional Food and Nutraceutical Products. Elsevier, pp. 1–28.

Kalra, E.K., 2003. Nutraceutical-definition and introduction. AAPS Pharm. Sci. 5 (3), 27–28.

Menrad, K., 2003. Market and marketing of functional food in Europe. J. Food Eng. 56 (2), 181–188.

Mirabella, N., Castellani, V., Sala, S., 2014. Current options for the valorization of food manufacturing waste: a review. J. Clean. Prod. 65, 28–41.

Mutalipassi, M., Esposito, R., Ruocco, N., Viel, T., Costantini, M., Zupo, V., 2021. Bioactive compounds of nutraceutical value from fishery and aquaculture discards. Foods 10 (7), 1495.

Naylor, R.W., Droms, C.M., Haws, K.L., 2009. Eating with a purpose: consumer response to functional food health claims in conflicting versus complementary information environments. J. Public Policy Market. 28 (2), 221–233.

Ohama, H., Ikeda, H., Moriyama, H., 2006. Health foods and foods with health claims in Japan. Toxicology (Amsterdam) 221 (1), 95–111.

Pagliaro, M., 2020. Italy's nutraceutical industry: a process and bioeconomy perspective into a key area of the global economy. Biofuels, Bioproducts Bioref. 14 (2), 180–186.

Pandey, M.M., Rastogi, S., Rawat, A.K.S., 2013. Indian traditional ayurvedic system of medicine and nutritional supplementation. Evidence-Based Complementary Alternative Med. 376327. https://doi.org/10.1155/2013/376327.

Payyappallimana, U., Venkatasubramanian, P., 2016. Exploring ayurvedic knowledge on food and health for providing innovative solutions to contemporary healthcare. Front. Public Health 4, 57. https://doi.org/10.3389/fpubh.2016.00057.

Rutsaert, P., Regan, Á., Pieniak, Z., McConnon, Á., Moss, A., Wall, P., Verbeke, W., 2013. The use of social media in food risk and benefit communication. Trends Food Sci. Technol. 30 (1), 84–91.

Santini, A., Novellino, E., 2017. To nutraceuticals and back: rethinking a concept. Food 6 (9), 74–77. doi:10.3390/foods6090074.

Stefan, N., Birkenfeld, A.L., Schulze, M.B., 2021. Global pandemics interconnected—obesity, impaired metabolic health and COVID-19. Nature Rev. Endocrinol. 17 (3), 135–149. https://doi.org/10.1038/s41574-020-00462-1.

Tobey Lauren, N., Manore Melinda, M., 2014. Social media and nutrition education: the food hero experience. J. Nutr. Education Behavior 46 (2), 128–133.
Varela-Candamio, L., Calvo, N., Novo-Corti, I., 2018. The role of public subsidies for efficiency and environmental adaptation of farming: A multi-layered business model based on functional foods and rural women. J. Clean. Prod. 183, 555–565.

CHAPTER 2

A short review on willingness to pay for novel food

Maurizio Canavari, Alessandra Castellini, Vilma Xhakollari
Department of Agricultural and Food Sciences, Alma Mater Studiorum-University of Bologna, Bologna, Italy

2.1 Introduction

The increasing world population pressures scientists and companies to introduce new food production practices (FAO, 2016). Thus, new developments in technology are seen as necessary to be introduced in the food production systems to facilitate and improve the impacts of the increasing food demand on the environment.

These advancements have introduced a new definition for food produced with modern technologies. In the European Union (EU) regulation, a "novel food" is defined as (1) a newly developed, innovative food; (2) a food produced using new technologies and production processes; or (3) a food that is or has been traditionally eaten outside of the EU and has not been consumed within the EU to a significant degree (McElhatton and Sobral, 2012; The European Parliament and the Council of the European Union, 2015). Nevertheless, this definition is true only within the EU, and what might be considered novel in the EU is not considered such in other parts of the world. Thus, finding a clear "novel food" definition is very difficult.

Considering these trends, it is necessary to understand the consumers' perception about these products, probably in different regions of the world, considering especially economic aspects such as willingness to pay for this category of products. Willingness to pay is a monetary measure of the utility or value perceived by individuals for a specific good/service/attribute. WTP for whole goods or, more often, for attributes, has been measured using various methods, such as contingent valuation, discrete choice experiments, experimental auctions. Insights from WTP measurement can be used to understand consumers' preferences and help companies design their pricing strategies for new products. Another important element to consider

Table 2.1 Process of the review.

Search	Articles	Screening	Final
Databases: Scopus (9 articles) Web of Science (10 articles) Econ papers (1 article) Science direct (161 articles) Ag econ search (12 articles) Query: "novel food" AND "willingness to pay" AND "consumer"	193 articles	No: Review papers Time limitation Duplicates Yes: Type of papers: academic jour- nals, conference proceedings, books, thesis, and dissertations Languages: English, Italian and Spanish Title and abstract: "novel food," "innovative," "artificial," "cultured," and "willingness to pay"	18 articles

is that WTP is being applied to many fields for estimating the importance perceived by consumers for a given good, service, or attribute.

The present chapter aims to understand the most important factors affecting the WTP by exploring the literature on novel food. We have considered only those articles studying economic aspects, excluding other relevant factors (e.g., psychological) or those focusing on purchase intentions without quantifying the willingness to pay (Table 2.1).

2.2 Methodology and data

The present review was conducted by running searches on five scientific literature databases (Scopus, Web of Science, EconPapers, AgEconSearch, and Science Direct), using the keywords (search query) "novel food," "willingness to pay," and "consumer." Since no previous reviews on this topic were found, the time range was open.

The main purpose of this search was to extract the available economic research on novel food. In total, 193 articles were identified from the database search. We conducted a screening process following these criteria:

- Articles from academic journals, conference proceedings, books, thesis.
- Materials published in English, Italian and Spanish language (languages spoken by the authors).
- Articles with the presence of the words "novel food," "innovative," "artificial," "cultured," and "willingness to pay" in their titles and abstracts.

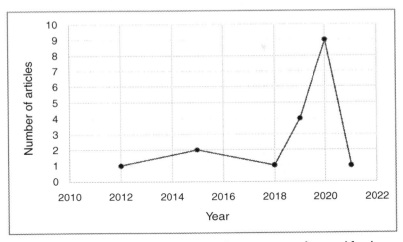

Fig. 2.1 *Number of articles published on the willingness to pay for novel food.*

After the screening, 18 articles were considered for review. Considering the limited number and the very diverse nature of the articles, in terms of products, technologies, and purpose, and in addition, the vague definition of "novel food," we did not conduct a systematic review.

The papers have been classified by region, product type, and production technology. Key results were evaluated and included in the analysis.

As Fig. 2.1 shows, despite the novel food regulation in the EU is dating back to 1997, most of the selected articles related to novel foods were published in recent years, especially in 2019 and 2020. It is expected that the number will increase more during the future years due to lifestyle changes and the policies followed by the EU. As shown in Fig. 2.2, most of the selected studies have been conducted in Europe (mainly in Italy) and the Americas (mainly in the USA).

The types of products analysed in the examined studies are very variable. Most of the studies analysed the acceptance of bakery and meat products produced mainly with proteins deriving from insects and enriched with functional ingredients. The interest in bakery products is consistent with an increasing trend of wheat-related allergies in western countries where 0.5%–9% of the population worldwide is affected by this allergy (Leonard and Vasagar, 2014). Regarding ruminant livestock (lamb and beef), the interest is in line with the fact that the demand for meat is expected to increase from 28 kg in 2005/2007 to 42 kg in 2050 in developing countries and from 80 to 91 kg in developed countries (Herrero et al., 2015). At

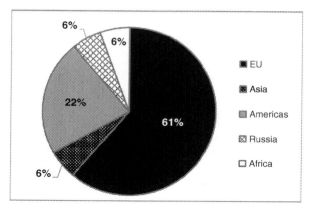

Fig. 2.2 *Country of origin of the articles.*

present, 80% of agricultural land is used for providing food for the animals (Herrero et al., 2015), and livestock is considered to have the highest impact on gas emissions (Clune et al., 2017). Thus, shifting towards alternative diets is deemed a way to mitigate climate change.

The following sections summarise the findings of the selected papers, considering separately consumer perception of novel food and the factors affecting their willingness to pay.

2.3 Consumers' perception of novel food

When first launched, innovation usually faces some skepticism, especially when dealing with food-related directly to people's well-being. To illustrate is worth mentioning the ban of genetically modified (GM) products in Europe. However, considering the future food system's challenges, especially due to the increasing population worldwide and climate change, innovative food-producing systems might be the only way to cope. Thus, considering the acceptance level of innovative food-producing systems from part of the consumers is crucial. Biondi and Camanzi (2020) found that consumers' willingness to buy is mainly affected by product perception and the individual's novelty-seeking orientation. In line with this finding, Grasso and Asioli (2020) found that participants were curious to try food produced with upcycled ingredients. In addition, a study from Ardebili and Rickertsen (2020) aimed at understanding how personality traits affect the Norwegian consumers' acceptance of three different GM products, GM soybean oil, GM-fed salmon, and GM salmon. It was observed that neuroticism[a] and conscientiousness[b] were associated with increased acceptance of the products. Other personal factors, such as socio-demographic characteristics, affect the acceptance of novel food. According to Van Loo et al. (2020), males, younger, and more highly educated individuals tend to have relatively stronger preferences for plant and lab-grown meat alternatives.

Nevertheless, it is relevant to mention that food and technology neophobia are limiting factors for increasing the market share of novel food and Millennials are not willing to buy food produced with upcycled ingredients (Coderoni and Perito, 2021). Since food neophobia is related to the avoidance of consuming new food, information might positively influence the acceptance of novel food. The literature also confirms this intuition. According to Bruschi et al. (2015), information about the enhancing characteristics of bread rolls and biscuits produced with purple wheat, naturally rich in anthocyanins, positively affected their acceptance over the conventional one even though the knowledge of the participants about purple wheat was low or absent. In line with this finding, Mancini and Antonioli (2020) show that positive information about cultured meat positively affects the perception of the product's nutritional and safety aspects. Another study on cultured meat found that even though a majority of the participants did not have information about artificial meat, after explaining what artificial meat is, the percentage of people not willing to buy the product decreased (Zhang et al., 2020). These results are supported also by a recent systematic review that found that public awareness influences the acceptance of cultured meat (Pakseresht et al., 2021).

But how to communicate information to the consumers? According to Coderoni and Perito (2021), introducing the environmental benefits of novel food positively impacts accepting food produced with upcycled ingredients. In line with this, when provided with information about the environment and technology, the percentage of participants not willing to buy any food produced with alternative proteins decreased (Van Loo et al., 2020). These results are also true for nonmeat products (Grasso and Asioli, 2020). CEOs of alternative meat companies state that plant-based proteins could bring an end to the world's hunger, but no clear scientific evidence supports these declarations (Van Eenennaam and Werth, 2021). Furthermore, alternative meat production faces many challenges, among

---

[a]A chronic level of emotional instability and proneness to psychological distress (Ardebili and Rickertsen, 2020).
[b]The tendency to be organized, responsible, and hardworking (Ardebili and Rickertsen, 2020).

which nutritional, organoleptic, and economic factors remain unresolved (Rubio et al., 2020). Thus, the quality of information remains a critical point to resolve since it might bring important consequences to the public health and economies.

2.4 Factors affecting willingness to pay for novel food

Setting the right price and understanding the WTP is crucial, especially for new products (Hofstetter et al., 2013).

Studies on insect-based food products have shown that high prices affect the WTP positively. In other words, consumers are willing to pay more for products with high tag prices than for those with a low tag price (Berger et al., 2018). This phenomenon suggests that, currently, insect-based food is perceived as a specialty and a luxury, status showing, elite good. In addition, de-Magistris et al. (2015) found that consumers are willing to pay a higher premium price for insect-based products with a nutritional health claim and logo. However, they are not willing to pay for a product with an insect shape or an insect on it. Moreover, the taste is another factor that experiences increases in the WTP for novel insect-based bakery products, but the peer effect has a greater influence than taste on WTP (Alemu and Olsen, 2020).

Studies on artificial meat found similar results. A study conducted in China found that 70% of the participants were willing to taste or purchase cultured meat and were willing to pay 2.2% more than conventional meat (Zhang et al., 2020). In addition, the literature has shown that personal characteristics also affect the WTP for alternative meat. According to Mancini and Antonioli (2020), the WTP premium price for cultured meat depends mainly on the intention to reduce meat consumption, studying or already to obtain a university degree, young adults (18–44 years old) considering themselves as familiar with cultured meat.

Like studies on meat, studies on bakery products also found that the way the information is presented affects the WTP for bread and biscuits enriched with functional properties (Bruschi et al., 2015). In line with this, Bhatt et al. (2020) found that participants are willing to pay less for the upcycled product compared to the conventional one. However, messaging can affect this choice, especially from a logical perspective rather than an emotional one. Finally, according to Grasso and Asioli (2020), WTP is mainly affected by price, carbon trust label, protein, and type of flour.

A summary of the factors mentioned above is shown in Fig. 2.3

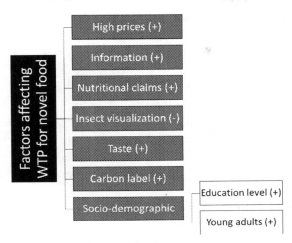

Fig. 2.3 *Factors affecting WTP for novel food.*

2.5 Conclusions and future research

This short review is aimed at understanding the state of the art about consumer preferences for novel food and other economic aspects related to these products. The number of articles focusing on economic aspects of a novel food is still very limited, and most of the studies have been conducted recently, especially in western countries. This finding might be in line with the fact that the Western diet relies more on meat proteins than other regions of the world, like Asia, where plant-based and insect-based proteins are more commonly included in the daily diet.

One important element to consider in future research is the definition of novel food. While there is a regulation in Europe that provides a clear definition of what novel food is, in other parts of the world, novel foods are defined differently or are not regulated. Hence, the lack of a clear and common understanding of the novel food concept makes it difficult to consistently describe and estimate the global market's size. A clear definition is necessary also for the fact that the number of articles considering economical aspects of novel food is increasing and it is expected to increase in the future due to the advancements in technologies applied for the food production and more sustainable eating habits from part of the consumers.

Regarding consumers' preferences, in general, it was noticed that consumers prefer conventional products over novel ones. However, when introduced with adequate information about nutritional and environmental aspects, their preference tends to switch towards more innovative products. This phenomenon is especially observed with young and highly educated individuals.

When carefully informed about novel foods, consumers tend to be willing to pay a premium price for novel food compared to the conventional counterpart. Thus, information is one of the key points to be considered in future research and measuring how and how much it affects consumers' preferences and WTP for novel food. Quality of information is another essential aspect to consider since the concept of novel food, although defined in the regulation, is still new in the consumers' vocabulary, and the risk of misunderstanding and the misuse of information might be quite relevant.

Research on novel food and its economic aspects is still limited despite growing interest. While some studies on meat and bakery products are available, studies on other food protein sources, like milk and/or eggs, are missing. This lack of research coverage is something to consider carefully in the future since in these product categories, the market for substitutes is already growing, and it is foreseeable that more firms will enter the novel food market in other food categories.

References

Alemu, M.H., Olsen, S.B., 2020. An analysis of the impacts of tasting experience and peer effects on consumers' willingness to pay for novel foods. Agribusiness 36 (4), 653–674. https://doi.org/10.1002/agr.21644.

Ardebili, A.T., Rickertsen, K., 2020. Personality traits, knowledge, and consumer acceptance of genetically modified plant and animal products. Food Qual. Preference 80 (May 2019), 103825. https://doi.org/10.1016/j.foodqual.2019.103825.

Berger, S., Christandl, F., Schmidt, C., Baertsch, C., 2018. Price-based quality inferences for insects as food. British Food J. 120 (7), 1615–1627. https://doi.org/10.1108/BFJ-08-2017-0434.

Bhatt, S., Ye, H., Deutsch, J., Ayaz, H., Suri, R., 2020. Consumers' willingness to pay for upcycled foods. Food Qual. Preference 86 (January), 104035. https://doi.org/10.1016/j.foodqual.2020.104035.

Biondi, B., Camanzi, L., 2020. Nutrition, hedonic or environmental? The effect of front-of-pack messages on consumers' perception and purchase intention of a novel food product with multiple attributes. Food Res. Int. 130 (December 2019), 108962. https://doi.org/10.1016/j.foodres.2019.108962.

Bruschi, V., Teuber, R., Dolgopolova, I., 2015. Acceptance and willingness to pay for health-enhancing bakery products—empirical evidence for young urban Russian consumers. Food Qual. Pref. 46, 79–91. https://doi.org/10.1016/j.foodqual.2015.07.008.

Clune, S., Crossin, E., Verghese, K., 2017. Systematic review of greenhouse gas emissions for different fresh food categories. J. Clean. Prod. 140, 766–783. https://doi.org/10.1016/j.jclepro.2016.04.082.

Coderoni, S., Perito, M.A., 2021. Approaches for reducing wastes in the agricultural sector. An analysis of Millennials' willingness to buy food with upcycled ingredients. Waste Manag. 126 (November 2020), 283–290. https://doi.org/10.1016/j.wasman.2021.03.018.

de-Magistris, T., Pascucci, S., Mitsopoulos, D., 2015. Paying to see a bug on my food: How regulations and information can hamper radical innovations in the European Union. British Food J. 117 (6), 1777–1792. https://doi.org/10.1108/BFJ-06-2014-0222.

FAO. (2016). Coping with Water Scarcity in Agriculture: a Global Framework for Action in a Changing Climate. FAO, Rome, Italy.

Grasso, S., Asioli, D., 2020. Consumer preferences for upcycled ingredients: a case study with biscuits. Food Qual. Preference 84 (January), 103951. https://doi.org/10.1016/j.foodqual.2020.103951.

Herrero, M., Wirsenius, S., Henderson, B., Rigolot, C., Thornton, P., Havlík, P., Gerber, P., 2015. Livestock and the environment: what have we learned in the past decade? Ann. Rev. Environ. Res. 40, 177–202. Vol. https://doi.org/10.1146/annurev-environ-031113-093503.

Hofstetter, R., Miller, K.M., Krohmer, H., Zhang, Z.J., 2013. How do consumer characteristics affect the bias in measuring willingness to pay for innovative products? J. Product Innovation Manag. 30 (5), 1042–1053. https://doi.org/10.1111/jpim.12040.

Leonard, M.M., Vasagar, B., 2014. US perspective on gluten-related diseases. Clinical Exp. Gastroenterol. 7 (1), 25–37. https://doi.org/10.2147/CEG.S54567.

Mancini, M.C., Antonioli, F., 2020. To what extent are consumers' perception and acceptance of alternative meat production systems affected by information? The case of cultured meat. Animals 10 (4). https://doi.org/10.3390/ani10040656.

McElhatton, A., & Sobral, P.J.A. (2012). Novel Technologies in Food Science: Their Impact on Products, Consumer Trends and the Environment. Springer, New York, NY. https://doi.org/10.1007/978-1-4419-7880-6

Pakseresht, A., Kaliji, S.A., Canavari, M., 2021. Review of factors affecting consumer acceptance of cultured meat. Appetite 170, 105829. https://doi.org/10.1016/j.appet.2021.105829.

Rubio, N.R., Xiang, N., Kaplan, D.L., 2020. Plant-based and cell-based approaches to meat production. Nature Commun. 11 (1), 1–11. https://doi.org/10.1038/s41467-020-20061-y.

The European Parliament and the Council of the European Union, 2015. Regulation (EU) 2015/2283 of the European Parliament and of the Council of 25 November 2015 on novel foods, amending Regulation (EU) No 1169/2011 of the European Parliament and of the Council and repealing Regulation (EC) No 258/97 etc. J. European Union 327 (258), 1–22.

Van Eenennaam, A.L., Werth, S.J., 2021. Animal board invited review: animal agriculture and alternative meats—learning from past science communication failures. Animal 15 (10), 100360. https://doi.org/10.1016/j.animal.2021.100360.

Van Loo, E.J., Caputo, V., Lusk, J.L., 2020. Consumer preferences for farm-raised meat, lab-grown meat, and plant-based meat alternatives: Does information or brand matter? Food Policy 95 (July), 101931. https://doi.org/10.1016/j.foodpol.2020.101931.

Zhang, M., Li, L., Bai, J., 2020. Consumer acceptance of cultured meat in urban areas of three cities in China. Food Control 118 (May), 107390. https://doi.org/10.1016/j.foodcont.2020.107390.

CHAPTER 3

Market-oriented methodologies that integrate the consumer into the functional foods new product development process: Part 1 contemporary approaches

Joe Bogue, Lana Repar
Department of Food Business and Development, Cork University Business School, University College Cork, Ireland

3.1 Introduction

The functional foods market represents a significant opportunity for food firms in terms of market growth, high levels of added value, brand differentiation, and the development of innovative products, closely aligned with dynamic consumer trends. In this chapter, we examine contemporary market-oriented approaches to the design and development of new functional foods. These approaches entail using methodologies that integrate the *voice of the consumer* into the early stages of the new product development (NPD) process, where concept definition occurs, and then throughout the process. The early design stages of the NPD process are important as multidisciplinary teams understand consumers' needs, and integrate the information generated into the design and development of new functional foods. The subsequent stages of NPD, such as prototyping, market validation, and product launch also significantly benefit from consumers' insights. Using market-oriented methodologies to generate insights for the early definition of the product concept can ultimately lead to more successful functional foods. The market research methodologies covered in this chapter include focus group discussions, ethnography, netnography, and semiotics. Each is outlined with a set of relevant business and market questions it can address and supported by examples. As will be seen from the case studies, when the methodologies are used on their own, or in combination, in the right

Case Studies on the Business of Nutraceuticals, Functional and Super Foods
DOI: https://doi.org/10.1016/B978-0-12-821408-4.00002-X
31

context, can inspire similar ground-breaking research into functional foods through the generation of invaluable new consumer insights.

3.2 New product development: Functional foods challenges

Developing new products is a knowledge-intensive process and requires in-depth knowledge of both products and consumers. It is a very complex and risky venture for food firms and it is generally accepted that 90% of all new food products fail within one year of launch (Fig. 3.1). The development of new functional foods, with specific functional ingredients, presents many marketing and technical challenges for product developers.

The factors that impact consumers' food choices are extremely complex, and food choice in relation to functional foods is even more complex, thus the development and marketing of functional foods is risky for firms. Consumer acceptance and purchase of functional foods is multidimensional and linked to factors such as (1) motivations to change dietary behaviour; (2) nutrition knowledge; (3) belief in the efficacy of the functional ingredients; (4) acceptance of the product carrier, such as whether it is dairy, water or juiced based; (5) age and socio-economic status of the consumer segment; and (6) the health status of the consumer. In addition, van Trijp and van Kleef (2008) highlighted that consumers hold an inherent tendency to approach (*neophilia*) and avoid (*neophobia*) new food products at the same time. Thus, those developing new functional foods need to generate accurate and relevant consumer information and use this information to drive the NPD process.

There is a wide range of marketing challenges to be overcome to successfully launching new functional foods, including (1) the health claims and consumer knowledge of the health benefits of ingredients; (2) consumer perceptions of functional foods versus dietary supplements; and (3) identifying consumer segments that pay a premium for functional foods. In addition, it is likely that a key target market for functional foods in future will be the ageing consumer segment. The global population aged 65 years or over reached 727 million in 2020, with the number of older persons expected to double again by 2050, when it is projected to amount to nearly 1.5 billion (United Nations, 2020). For this consumer segment, it will be important to understand their requirements, particularly regarding: the belief in the health claims that are made by functional food firms; the extent to which they believe in the efficacy of functional foods; and whether those foods are seen as part of a healthy diet.

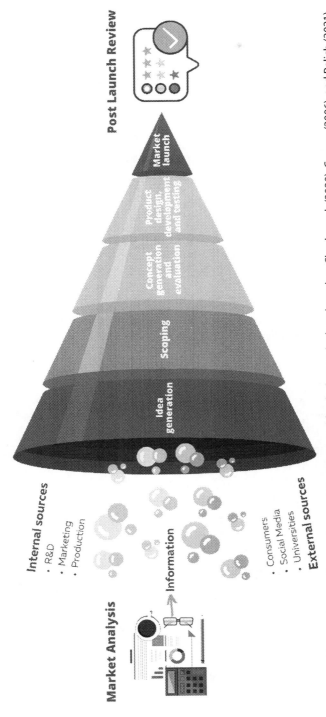

Fig. 3.1 *New product development process for functional foods. Source:* Authors based on Chesbrough (2020), Cooper (2006), and Relich (2021). Created using Canva Pro.

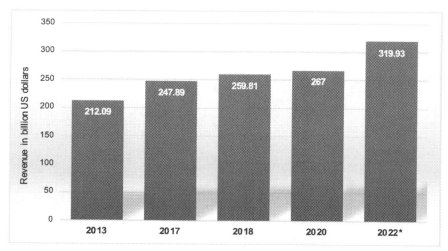

Fig. 3.2 *Fortified/functional food market revenue generated worldwide (2013–22).*
Source: Wunsch (2020). Note: the figures for 2022 are forecasted.

3.3 Challenging marketing myopia: Co-creating new functional foods with consumers

The revenue generated by the functional food market globally is forecasted to increase substantially, from around US$212 billion in 2013 to US$320 billion by 2022 (Fig. 3.2). However, there are large numbers of food firms, including blue-chip firms, that have launched functional foods that have failed and, so the question becomes: How do firms develop more successful market-oriented functional foods?

Corporate marketing myopia characterises firms as those that have neglected to appreciate the value of an institutional, stakeholder, and societal orientation (Podnar and Balmer, 2021). In consumer food markets, firms often focus more on selling rather than seeking an in-depth understanding of their consumers. Therefore, firms should continually identify consumer needs, now and into the future, rather than just producing and selling products in the short term. In addition, new approaches to idea generation, such as *open innovation* and *design crowdsourcing*, are ideally suited to incorporate external ideas from consumers, and online communities have become an important source of knowledge and ideas (Chesbrough, 2020; Garcia Martinez, 2017).

Narver and Slater (1990) proposed that market orientation helped create the necessary behaviours within an organization that offered superior value for consumers and this, in turn, benefited a firm's business performance. Thus, it is a business philosophy where the focus is on identifying consumer needs or wants and meeting them. When a firm has a market-oriented approach, it focuses on designing and selling goods and services that satisfy consumer needs in order to be profitable (Narver and Slater, 1990). From this, a market-oriented approach suggests that a business reacts to what consumers want. The decisions taken are based around information about consumers' needs and wants, rather than what the business thinks is right for the consumer.

Market orientation is a key to new product success and consists of various components, but essentially seeks to stay close to the consumer during the NPD process, particularly at the early design stages, and use advanced market research methodologies to understand the consumer. It is about knowledge management and using relevant information from the consumer, in terms of refining existing products and developing new products, to meet, and exceed, consumer needs. Market orientation is particularly relevant to developing functional foods, where innovations are often driven by science and technology (Push) and developing producer value, rather than based on consumer demands (Pull) and developing consumer value (Sorenson and Bogue, 2009).

Market-oriented firms are more likely to be profitable and successful at developing new products. The key components of the market orientation grouping linked to NPD success are degree of product superiority (measured from consumers' point of view); the amount and/or frequency of contact with market/consumers during development; degree of upfront marketing; representation of the marketing function in the development process; the amount of market and/or competitor knowledge; use of advanced market research methodologies; test marketing; and prototype tests with consumers (Harmsen, 1994). In this chapter, we examine the use of methodological approaches that generate *voice of the consumer*, to inform the process of developing new functional foods.

The market-oriented approach to NPD places the consumer as co-creator or co-designer in the NPD process. However, it is often argued there are low levels of market-orientation within the food sector (Harmsen et al., 2000). For functional foods, with the inherent marketing and technical challenges that they present, particularly in terms of marketing science to consumers, a market-oriented approach to developing new products becomes more important.

3.4 Methodological approaches for consumer insights

Successful product developers understand in-depth what consumers need, what they do not need, and their motivations to purchase specific foods or brands. In many cases where functional foods have failed in the market-place, the product concept was not clearly understood by consumers. There is a wide range of market research methodological approaches that can be used to generate information from the consumer. For functional foods, these methodologies can be used for ideation and to generate information on novel ideas; to gauge levels of acceptance of new functional foods; to understand the perceived benefits of ingredients; to evaluate knowledge of the health benefits of ingredients science; and to examine attribute trade-offs, occasions of use, desired sensory profiles, design of packaging, and effective marketing messaging.

It is important to emphasise that, for a thorough and in-depth approach to NPD, detailed secondary research should precede any primary research. Secondary research can be focused on different aspects. For example, a sys-tematic review can reveal consumer insights and specialist knowledge on a product's features. Exploring the most recent consumer trends can unearth valuable tips on potential future directions. In addition, using statistics from search engines is surging and one of the applications in NPD is to look for key search words/phrases related to a trend, ingredient or product, to understand what consumers are interested in. This can often reveal infor-mation on novel ingredients, their uses, and related health claims.

3.4.1 Focus group discussions

3.4.1.1 History and recent developments

Focus group discussions are one of the most frequently used methods of data collection in market research. This methodology creates a unique opportunity to explore a relationship between consumers' beliefs, life-style, and influences, and the food purchase decision. The origins of focus groups are found in the work of Bogardus who in 1926 conducted social psychological research and described group interviews (Liamputtong, 2011). Later in the 1950s, Merton et al. (1956) used focus group discus-sions to examine reactions to wartime propaganda and first used the term "focus group". In the 1950s and 1960s, the methodology was used to study consumer attitudes to advertisements, TV programmes and movies, and perceptions of new products and services (Goffin et al., 2010). Up to the late 1970s, focus groups were mainly used in market research, and in the

1990s the methodology has been adopted and used by social scientists in the areas such as education, health, communication, media, and sociology (Wilkinson, 2020).

There is a recent "resurrection" of the importance of a *discussion* and its meaning in the focus groups. The interaction and group dynamics between the participants are so valuable that Belzile and Öberg (2012), Farnsworth and Boon (2010), and Halkier (2010) argued that they should be made a conscious and explicit design decision, and that there is a need to better understand social interactions and group dynamics. This is particularly important when it comes to functional foods as the group interaction can reveal hidden insights on *how*, and *why*, certain functional foods are accepted by consumers. Furthermore, the increased application of information and communication technologies in consumer studies paved the way for some notable advantages. Online focus groups can reduce the costs for firms developing new foods, assist in faster market data collection, remove challenges related to timing and location, allow recruitment of more demographically and geographically diverse participants with lower dropout rates, encourage participation and self-disclosure due to visual anonymity and psychological distance, and generate idea diversity that is comparable to in-person focus groups (Halliday et al., 2021; Reid and Reid, 2005; Richard et al., 2020). Brown et al. (2021) found that online focus groups worked well with younger consumers, while Colom (2021) proposed using new social media technologies, such as WhatsApp, which would promote familiarity and inclusivity and encourage more group deliberation.

3.4.1.2 Focus group procedure, advantages, and challenges

A focus group discussion represents a qualitative approach, where the aim is to bring together purposely selected participants to discuss particular topics. It usually involves six to eight participants from similar backgrounds, or shared experiences, related to a specific area under research (Hennik, 2014; Liamputtong, 2011). Through a carefully planned series of discussions, researchers gather rich, contextual data to gain an in-depth understanding of consumers' perceptions, attitudes, and habits, in a permissive, nonthreatening environment (Krueger and Casey, 2015). Unlike quantitative approaches, focus groups provide many opportunities to probe the question *Why?*, which is essential for understanding in-depth participants' reasoning and corresponding actions. The key advantage of this method is a facilitated discussion taking place among the participants. While such discussion requires a skilful facilitator, it has the power to capture a myriad of different layers of consumer behaviour: from consensus among the participants, confrontations, opposite opinions and values, to the phenomenon of evolving attitudes which can be the result of either a fruitful discussion, or peer pressure. To a certain degree, focus groups have the potential to replicate real-life situations, where consumers are exposed to competing functional foods and various social influences that could ultimately drive their purchase decision. Other advantages of focus groups include the generation of complex information quickly and at relatively low cost.

While focus groups have many advantages, this method is not without challenges. Focus group discussion questions need to be phrased to encourage discussion among the participants, avoiding *Yes* or *No* responses. A discussion guide needs to be designed in a way to allow the discussion to naturally follow its own course. The facilitator plays a key, but discrete role, in a focus group discussion. The key challenge for the facilitator is to simultaneously ensure a solid debate occurs, cover the key questions, and monitor that the data recorded are useful to address the research problem. The reality of focus groups is that participants are likely to have different personalities. Some of them are very open and suitable for a discussion-type scenario, but others might have difficulties accepting other participants' opinions, or do not like to share their thoughts (Fig. 3.3).

Once all data are collected, the recordings are usually transcribed and then analysed. Unlike quantitative data analysis where various software perform complex calculations, qualitative data analysis is inherently subjective and requires time and space to evolve into relevant and trustworthy material. Software like *NVivo*, *ATLAS.ti*, and *Quirkos* assist in organising the transcripts and allow the researcher to visualise and group the codes and create nodes, which is the foundation for developing categories and themes. Qualitative data analysis is often performed using a content or thematic analysis, although there are many other options such as the interpretative phenomenological analysis or grounded theory, but they are strongly embedded in the accompanying theory. Classical content analysis is focused on quantifying the collected data by examining the content and capturing the frequency and patterns of a term or a phrase (Savin-Baden and Howell Major, 2013). This type of analysis can be useful, for example, for unravelling frequent words, positive or negative, used to describe functional foods. Thematic analysis represents an iterative process of noticing patterns and constructing emerging themes that contain the content and meaning of patterns (Braun and Clarke, 2006), relevant for in-depth understanding of more abstract constructs related to functional foods.

Indifferent
- Do not really have an opinion
- Do not contribute much
- Wish they were somewhere else

Confused
- Confused about the concept of the discussion
- Probably never participated before
- Might get the question wrong

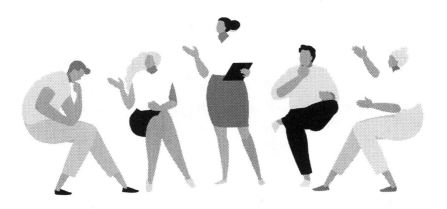

Quiet & shy
- Do not like to talk in the group
- Afraid to express their opinion
- Might agree with others just so they do not have to give their opinion

Bossy
- Think they run the show
- Might give you instructions
- Might correct others

Loud & opinionated
- Think they know it all
- Have something to say always
- Might openly criticise others

Fig. 3.3 *Types of participants in a focus group discussion. Source:* Authors. Created using Canva Pro. Art elements: artbesouro.

3.4.1.3 Focus group in the context of new product development and functional foods

A focus group works particularly well in the exploratory phase of NPD. Some of the areas where focus groups are useful include: exploring new ingredients, formats, and flavours; packaging; usage occasions; reformulation; branding; marketing messaging; and identifying the appropriate target market. Consumer insights from focus group often serve as a starting point for early concept designs, helping to navigate between product features that participants accept or reject, and intention to purchase. Participants often have limited knowledge of the most recent developments in food trends, and their suggestions are likely to be narrow and bounded by current experiences. Hence, optimal results for NPD occur when consumer insights are integrated with information from the *voice of the expert*, such as food scientists or technologists. Combined together, their insights offer an invaluable pool of information for firms. Another stage where the application of focus groups is essential is prototyping. This phase usually follows once several key features of a new product have been identified and focus group participants are given an opportunity to express their opinions on different variations of a product. A useful approach is to recruit representatives of the potential target market since a discussion at this stage will result in understanding participants' acceptance of the new functional food attributes.

3.4.1.4 Selected business and market issues that can be addressed through focus groups

- Do consumers understand the product concept and is the carrier a logical fit?
- Does the product concept fit with consumers' daily buying and consumption habits?
- How do consumers compare the new product versus competitors' products?
- Do consumers accept the ingredient and do they understand the health claims?
- How do we develop our marketing strategy with our target market (4Ps: product, price, place, and promotion)?
- Do consumers prefer a familiar or a new brand? Does the health benefit fit with the brand image?

Box 3.1   More than just a function? Using focus groups to unpack deeper meanings

The way consumers understand the link between their wellbeing and functional foods is not often obvious. Conroy et al. (2021) explored how consumers perceive the complex construct of wellbeing, in the context of functional foods, using among others, eight focus group discussions with 48 contemporary Chinese consumers. The focus groups lasted between 90 and 120 min. and were audio-recorded. They were conducted in person using a semi-structured interview guide and a bilingual researcher, an English-speaking researcher, and a professional translator. The presence of two researchers enhanced the integrity and trustworthiness of the collected data and enabled triangulation to minimise researcher biases. Participants were recruited through purposeful sampling and inclusion/exclusion criteria set to identify information-rich individuals. The participants varied according to gender, health concerns, income, and occupation and were grouped based on age: younger (25–40) and older (41–55). Thematic analysis was used to analyse the collected data, and the findings were presented using pseudonymised quotations to capture the rich views and experiences of participants. Participants demanded provenance, which was easily identifiable from the label, and heuristic cues on what health improvement, and how quickly, the product would offer them. Understanding the target market, where consumers seek information, and what signals are being sought, was highlighted as important marketing information that could increase sales. Nevertheless, the most critical finding was that consumers seek to take control over their wellbeing, so marketing messaging should be created with this in mind. This study showed how focus groups revealed invaluable deeper meanings and expectations that consumers had regarding functional foods.

Case study based on: Conroy et al. (2021).

3.4.1.5 Selected steps in conducting a focus group to explore functional foods

1. Research current trends on functional foods related to consumer needs.
2. Where does the functional food fit in the NPD process (e.g., idea generation or testing and validation)?
3. Define the problem that needs to be addressed.
4. Develop an Interview Guide with a set of questions and probes to guide the discussion. Aim for 45–90 min discussions and identify props: images, slides, or prototypes.
5. Pilot the Interview Guide and make any necessary edits.
6. Recruit 6–8 participants per focus group.
7. Prepare audio and/or video equipment and secure a suitable location.
8. Conduct the focus groups until information saturation is achieved.
9. Record, make notes, notice group dynamics, and any valuable detail.
10. Transcribe the discussions.
11. Code the transcripts, compare and contrast all the focus groups and develop the relevant themes.
12. Report on the key findings and answer the research question(s).

3.4.2 Ethnography
3.4.2.1 History and recent developments

Ethnography is a qualitative research method central to knowing the world from the standpoint of its social relations and is relevant wherever people are relevant. It is predicated on the diversity of culture and involves hands-on, on-the-scene learning (Princeton, 2021). According to Petty et al. (2012), ethnography examines shared patterns of behaviour, beliefs, and language. One distinctive characteristic of ethnography is the focus on direct participant observation for an extended period. Therefore, it is a highly useful methodology for addressing a range of research questions within the NPD process. For example, product developers can obtain new consumer insights by observing consumers in their natural habitat and how they engage with, and use, products. In terms of functional foods, this includes how, and when, a consumer uses a product, what they use it for and how they engage with the product's packaging and portion size.

Traditionally, ethnography as a methodological tool has been central to anthropology, but it recently gained more interest in consumer research (Valentin and Gómez-Corona, 2018; Pountney and Marić, 2021). The beginning of the ethnographic methodology can be traced back to the period between the late 19th and early 20th centuries. It is generally accepted that Malinowski (1922) was the first to systematically describe the methodological principles underpinning ethnography in his 2-year-long study of native people in the Trobriands (New Guinea). Modern ethnography has changed, particularly in the way the study "subjects" are now considered as "partners and collaborators", as well as the adoption of new technologies (Lamphere, 2018; Taylor, 2017). Ethnography has been increasingly utilised to gather consumer-centric knowledge to assist marketers in understanding the socio–cultural dynamics of marketplace behaviour and inform marketing strategies and tactics, products and service development, and corporate strategy processes (Moisander et al., 2020). Recent developments, such as rapid ethnographies (RE), where research is carried over a short, compressed, or intensive period to capture key experiences and practices, are likely to increase the use of this methodology in consumer research (Vindrola-Padros, 2021).

3.4.2.2 Ethnographic study procedure, advantages, and challenges

Key features of ethnography include: a strong emphasis on exploring the nature of a particular social phenomenon; a tendency to work primarily with "unstructured data"; investigation of a small number of cases (perhaps even just one case) in detail; an analysis of data that involves explicit interpretation of the meanings and functions of human actions; and the product of this analysis takes the form of verbal descriptions and explanations (Reeves et al., 2008). Ethical conduct and respect for the participants at all times is a central consideration of this methodology. In marketing research, an ethnographic approach is a vehicle for gaining consumer insights by exploring patterns of consumption and *what*, *why*, and *how* people consume products and relate with a brand (Estey, 2019). An ethnographic study involves three main stages: (1) preparation for the study, including extensive desk research to frame the study subject(s) and studied phenomenon; (2) recruitment and immersion in the life of consumers that involves collecting different types of data (e.g., observations, interviews, audio-visual artefacts, and notes); and (3) thorough analysis and report of the key findings. Since an ethnographic study is likely to yield different types of data, this must be reflected in the chosen analysis. The goal is to bring together all information in a meaningful way to tell and interpret a story of the studied phenomenon.

The value of practical information on, for example, the occasion of use of functional foods is very beneficial, and this type of snapshot of consumer behaviour can rarely be achieved by other methodologies. Another advantage is that by observing consumers, developers can learn more about their own product and identify (1) which features work well, (2) what needs to improve, and even (3) which functional foods should be developed. Nonetheless, ethnography is a time-consuming, costly, and complex method. It relies on consumers' willingness to be observed for a long period and prior knowledge is needed to appropriately collect, analyse and interpret different types of data. In addition, the findings might not be applicable for wider consumer segments, unless a representative number of study subjects were carefully selected to represent the key characteristics of each consumer segment, including different socio-demographic circumstances and geographical locations.

3.4.2.3 Ethnography in the context of new product development and functional foods

Ethnography is mostly suitable for the later stages of NPD, when a functional food prototype is available and consumers can use it in everyday situations. There are two situations where this methodology particularly excels. First, ethnography can be used to understand consumers' low acceptance of existing functional foods by observing why consumers fail to opt for them, which could result in product redesign and greater market success. Second, observing how, and when, consumers use a new prototype, such as the meal occasion, or what foods they combine it with, produces critical insights for designing and marketing functional foods. Valuable information can be gathered in cases where (1) a household or a close group of subjects interact simultaneously with a functional food or (2) where those in single-person households consume it, as this more accurately represents real-life situations and marketers can better understand different group dynamics, personal motivations, and obstacles.

3.4.2.4 Selected business and market issues that can be addressed through ethnography

- How consumers prepare and use products?
- In which occasions and settings do consumers use products?
- Is the packaging user-friendly?
- Is there too little/too much in the portion size?
- What are the alternative ways in which the product could be used?
- Which other age, or lifestyle groups, could use the product?

Box 3.2   Consumer Immersion: how ethnography can address the needs of the elderly segment and food intolerant consumers

A key target market for functional foods is elderly consumers, who may consume them for ongoing health conditions or to prevent a specific illness. The elderly market is often called *the market of all markets* and, globally, 16% of population will be a member of this extremely heterogeneous group aged 65 or over by 2050, with more complicated buying behaviours than other generations (United Nations, 2020). However, there are few food products, if any, in markets *specifically* targeted only at elderly consumers and we know very little about the food preferences of this consumer group. Ethnographic research is a very useful way of understanding the role functional foods will play in the diets of elderly consumers. The benefit of using ethnographic research was shown very effectively by Clarks Shoes when their design team developed a new active walking boot using an ethnographic research approach. They interviewed walkers in national parks in the UK to understand what consumers meant by *comfort* as they set about designing a new hiking boot. They did this, rather than only conducting desk research, and went on to develop a market-leading hiking boot design based on consumer insights by using the consumer as a codesigner in the innovation process (Goffin et al., 2010). If we apply this ethnographic approach to the elderly consumer market, product developers can interview elderly consumers as they use food products, for example, a new ready meal with functional ingredients and the challenges they face with these products: ease of opening; portion size; product health claims and ingredients; meal occasions and other factors. This information can be built into the design of functional foods and help integrate consumers' articulation of issues into the NPD process. Both technical and marketing personnel can be present, or can review interviews, to see how the information can be interpreted to understand elderly consumers and their needs, in a setting that follows their daily routine, to design functional foods that may be more likely to gain acceptance by this segment.

In addition, an ethnographic approach is useful when developing gluten-free foods. Lewis and Mehmet (2021) used an autoethnographic study to explore the challenges of a group traveling in rural New Zealand with a gluten intolerance. One the six-day trip most of the meals (except breakfast) were consumed at restaurants. Preidentified themes of interest were set up before the trip: (1) food service providers' response to special food requirements; (2) emotional responses before, during, and after food purchase; and (3) factors influencing food selection and purchase behaviour. One author documented his experience in-situ, or shortly after the experience, through written notes, audio notes using a smartphone, and photos of venues and menus. The findings highlighted that this individual's food intolerance resulted in the avoidance of certain food categories and a low spend within the rural community. Autoethnography enabled a peek into the personal, vivid, and sometimes painful experience of a potential consumer with specific dietary requirements, and emphasised the need for appropriate signage pointing to food alternatives. In this context, the methodology provided invaluable insights into a consumer's day-to-day behaviour, which helps functional food firms to better understand what type of products they could include in their product portfolio (e.g., convenient travel size packaging), how to market them (e.g., clear gluten-free messaging), what channels to use (e.g., offering snacks in restaurants) and how to ensure that consumers do not feel isolated, or different, due to their food intolerances (e.g., use dynamic and "positive" packaging that emphasises benefits).

Case study based on: Lewis and Mehmet (2021).

3.4.2.5 Selected steps in conducting an ethnographic study to explore functional foods

1. Research the current trends on functional foods related to how consumers use these and similar products.
2. Where does the functional food fit in the NPD process (e.g., idea generation or testing and validation)?
3. Define the problem that needs to be addressed.
4. Clearly define the subject(s) you will be observing.
5. Decide on the duration, setting, researcher's role, and the data analysis.
6. Obtain ethical approval for the study.
7. Conduct your ethnographic study with the identified subject(s), within the set time and the setting, with utmost respect and, depending on the researcher's role, with more or less involvement.
8. Take extensive notes throughout the study, including audio, video, photographs, and sketches or diagrams that will later assist in reconstructing the subject(s) behaviour in relation to functional foods.

9. Conclude the study, reflect and analyse your materials.

10. Report on the key findings and answer the research question(s).

3.4.3 Netnography

3.4.3.1 History and recent developments

Simply put, netnography is ethnography applied in the virtual world and its evolution can be attributed to the internet and the profound impact it has on ethnography and the social sciences (Gobo and Cellini, 2021). It is a methodology that adapts the known participant–observation ethnographic procedures to study online culture and communities with an aim to obtain understandings of peoples' experiences from online social interaction and content (Kozinets, 2015, 2010). Coined in 1997 by Kozinets, this new methodology is gaining momentum. Netnography found its initial application in the marketing and consumer behaviour domain, although other sociological fields are also adopting this approach: from research on gambling practices, military and healthcare, to banking, tourism, and skincare (Kozinets, 2021). As various online communities, also called *e-tribes*, are established daily and cover specific member interests, netnography is a tool for gathering and interpreting online information.

Netnography itself is only one of the more recently developed methodologies that use an ethnographic approach in the online world. Although terms such as *virtual ethnography* (Hine, 2020), *online ethnography,* or *digital ethnography* (Caliandro, 2018 and Pink et al., 2015) are often used interchangeably, it is important to understand their subtle but important differences. For example, online ethnography might have less strict requirements and hence could be suitable for a firm's internal research, but a netnographic study requires deeper knowledge of the epistemological background, the role of the researcher, and the analysis.

3.4.3.2 Netnographic study procedure, advantages, and challenges

Through the means of netnography, a researcher will usually gather longer, or shorter, chunks of text or images created by community members on a specific topic via blogs, fora, dedicated websites, or social media. By combining data from multiple online channels (e.g., fora and social media), a researcher can gather significant amounts of data in a relatively short period of time. Depending on the researchers' needs, experiences and the preferences, there are four main types of netnographic research (Kozinets, 2015). In autonetnography, the researcher gathers the least amount of data but is personally invested in the research and unravels the "truths" of others through her/his own experience. Humanist netnography gathers manageable amounts of data and is focused on amplifying positive change through carefully selected curated stories, which are then shared with other netnographers and the wider audience. Symbolic netnography is very common and it seeks to collect considerable amounts of data from various sites, cultures, and groups in order to translate the way they operate as different values, practices, and rituals. For business research, digital netnography is probably the most interesting, as the researcher collects large amounts of data to gain a comprehensive and representative overview of a phenomenon, which often allows quantification of collected data.

A netnographic study involves (1) detailed planning and introspection, (2) community identification and selection, (3) entrée strategy, observation, and data collection, and (4) analysis, interpretation and reporting. Once data are gathered, it needs to be collated and prepared for the analysis and process, which might include *combining* to develop "pattern code", *quantifying* and/or *charting* (Kozinets, 2021). Netnography captures online data which usually follow a common thread, and it differs from other qualitative methodological approaches, such as focus groups and interviews, as it usually does not provide the answers to a facilitator's direct question. Therefore, the coding process is critical to this approach. Ethics-related issues are relevant for any netnographic research, which reminds us of its connection with ethnography.

Although still not mainstream, netnography has been used increasingly for several reasons. First, new opportunities for firms that the Internet and social media brought in the last two decades require a novel approach if they are to capture consumers' preferences online. Netnography enables gathering insights from online consumers as it utilises the immense ever-growing data supplied by consumers. Second, the new currency in today's business world is consumer data. Third, netnography bridges the key challenge of the ethnographic research process, that is, the lengthy recruitment and spending time with participants in a bounded geographical area. The opportunities for using netnography are increasing as society is becoming more vocal on the Internet. However, netnography is becoming underpinned by epistemological and theoretical elements, and while this enhances the trustworthiness and acceptance of this methodology in academic spheres, it risks abandonment in more practical business-like research. An example of this is the difference in a description of how to undertake a netnographic study: in 2010, Kozinets outlined five steps, which became a complex 12 step procedure in 2015. In addition, general confusion over the differences between netnography and online or virtual ethnography further threaten to erase the uniqueness and user-friendliness of netnography.

3.4.3.3 Netnography in the context of the new product development and functional foods

The use of netnography is appropriate at different stages of NPD, but perhaps the most effective utilisation of this methodology is for (1) generating and scoping new ideas and (2) feedback on existing products, with the emphasis on potential redesign or innovation. For example, focused monitoring of selected websites, fora, and social media outlets can result in identifying new ingredients, packaging, and marketing messaging to be used for new functional foods. In addition, exploring in what context online communities mention and comment on functional foods, as well as what they like and dislike about them, can inform strategic marketing decisions, whether to give an existing product a makeover or develop a new, improved offering.

3.4.3.4 Selected business and market issues that can be addressed through netnography

- What are the key health and lifestyle concerns of specific online communities?
- What do online communities say about functional foods? What are their expectations?
- What innovations do online communities suggest?
- How would a functional food fit the needs of a specific community?
- How does a functional food feature in social media (e.g., occasion of use and time of the day)?
- What type of content is optimal for promoting functional foods online?

Box 3.3   Closing the net? Capturing online consumer information

Cong et al. (2019) utilised netnography to explore Chinese consumers' perceptions of functional foods. The study focused on one of the biggest issues in China: air pollution. It identified the key attributes consumers expected from functional foods, designed to assist in the recovery from the impact of pollution on health. The authors used the commercial internet search engine *Baidu*, and its keyword analysis tool, to identify the searching behaviour of users in the context of air pollution between 2013 and 2017. The most frequently searched terms *Fog & smog* and *PM2.5* (a term related to pollution levels) were then typed separately into *Baidu* and the top 10 sites' results were explored to identify relevant social network sites. A total of seven social network sites used the two terms and four sites were selected based on preset criteria: (1) publicly available without membership or password protection; (2) provide discussions on air pollution; (3) written in Chinese; and (4) contained both search terms. Based on the relevance and popularity of the discussion and taking into consideration only discussions containing comments with more than 10 "Likes", the authors selected a total of 145 discussions and around 1200 comments. Data were analysed by developing nodes and related themes using NVivo 11. Some of the benefits Chinese consumers expected from functional foods were to boost their immunity, target the adverse impact of air pollution on the respiratory system, moisten lungs, and to supply micronutrients. In this case, the netnographic approach provided: (1) detailed insights on consumers' key concerns related to health and lifestyle and (2) "undisturbed" and relevant information on what consumers expect from functional foods which, as shown in the study, can be related to the environment-specific conditions of consumers' habitats. By matching consumers' expectations and addressing their concerns, functional foods can become even more successful.

Ofstehage (2021) used a digital ethnographic methodology to reveal what functional food consumption represented to consumers. This 14-month study captured information on Soylent from online communities such as Reddit fora, Twitter posts, podcasts, YouTube videos, public posts, and marketing. Soylent is a functional drinkable meal, a controversial *future food*, where five servings per day promise to meet a person's nutrient requirements. It is an example of an antifood that focuses on delivering highly effective nutrition but removes any connection with food history, preparation, enjoyment, or social sharing. This is best captured in the brand's tagline *Let us take a few things off your plate* (Soylent, 2021). Ofstehage (2021) found that the taste of Soylent was of little consequence, the texture was unpleasant and the flavours unremarkable. This study revealed that the consumption of Soylent barely extended beyond the mechanics of eating and represented a means to an end for work-focused consumers. The product fitted in with their busy lifestyles and supported convenience, efficiency, and dedication to their work. The study also provoked a question: *How "functional" should functional foods be?*

Case study based on: Cong et al. (2019) and Ofstehage (2021).

3.4.3.5 Selected steps in conducting a netnographic study for functional foods

1. Research the current trends on functional foods related to online communities.
2. Where does the functional food fit in the NPD process (e.g., idea generation or testing and validation)?
3. Define the problem that needs to be addressed.
4. Decide on which of the four types of netnography research best suits your study and the most appropriate analysis.
5. Define your field (e.g., the person, the group, the website) and the size of the field (e.g., one or multiple websites).

6. Decide on the researcher's role (e.g., minimum or maximum involvement).
7. Decide on the time period for the netnographic study (if relevant).
8. Obtain ethics approval, as well as permission from the firm, blogging website, community, or individuals to collect, analyse, use and publish the targeted public data. This step is critical and no study should commence before all permissions have been obtained.
9. Store the data. Analyse data based on their nature, for example, statistical analysis for the QUAN data and a thematic or content analysis for the QUAL data.
10. Report on the key findings and answer the research question(s).

3.4.4 Semiotics

3.4.4.1 History and recent developments

Semiotics is an investigation into how meaning is created and communicated. Its origins lie in the academic study of how signs and symbols, visual and linguistic, create meaning. Bignell (2002, p. 1) defines semiotics as *a way of analysing meanings by looking at the signs (like words, for instance, but also pictures, symbols etc.) which communicate meanings.* This can convey meaning from a brand or functional food packaging, and when designing and marketing functional foods this methodology can play a significant role in attracting consumers initially and then encouraging repeat purchases. Packaging is a key attribute of a product in terms of value proposition and the meanings that it communicates. A brand is all about communication. According to Arning (2020), semiotics seeks to study meaning and communication and a brand owner must know the cues embedded in pack design. These cues include language on the packs, materials, colours, logos, crests, typology, and symbols. Four main uses of semiotic methodology in modern package design involve brand understanding, brand inspiration, brand evaluation, and brand intelligence (Arning, 2020).

3.4.4.2 Semiotics procedure, advantages, and challenges

A semiotic methodology involves analysis through a semiotic sort. In this case, if a firm was developing a new functional juice beverage, it would electronically gather all similar products in the category. The firm would then get consumers to interpret the meaning from logos, colours, and design on the packaging, and create new functional juice beverage packaging, based on the outcomes of the consumer insight piece of work. The firm can then put together a mock-up concept of the new pack design and then go back to consumers to see whether the packaging gives the intended meanings in its design brief including colours, brand design, pack shape, font, health claim, and logos.

Box 3.4   Semiotics and packaging design for functional foods

One of the key identified factors for the successful launch and differentiation of functional foods is through packaging design which should emphasize convenience, indulgence and wellness, and not rely on the health benefit as a sole point of difference (Mellentin, 2014). Bogue and Troy (2016) used semiotics to develop new functional beverages that would appeal to a general market and to specific consumer groups. They showed how semiotics could be used to develop a new functional beverage in a category that was ultra-competitive and overcrowded with many undifferentiated product offerings. The aim of the semiotic analysis was to see what colours, logos, and designs and health symbols, would appeal to each group. They initially analysed all the prominent competitors' packaging on the market and then used the information to get consumers to see what meanings they would attribute to various visual stimuli in order to develop packaging for a new functional beverage. The key findings from the semiotic analysis were that certain colours were associated with healthy beverages. In addition, the inclusion of specific images enhanced the overall perception of increased health and wellness of functional beverages. The semiotic analysis showed the important role that consumers can play in the marketing of functional beverages and that certain colours (white, green, and yellow/orange) were synonymous with healthy beverages and specific images (healthy hearts, wheat shafts) added to the perception of health and wellness.

Case study based on: Bogue and Troy (2016).

A semiotic analysis benefits functional foods' developers in terms of positioning and communicating the product attributes, both intrinsic and extrinsic, and potential health benefits as well as the positioning of the brand. Some advantages of designing packaging with consumers include: (1) understanding what matters to consumers and what meanings they associate with certain signs; (2) identifying clearer marketing messaging; (3) using colours, symbols, and shapes that are not confusing, and (4) consistently positioning brands. Recruitment of target market representatives might be time-consuming and challenging, but it is important when conducting a semiotic study as the packaging needs to be designed with specific consumers in mind (e.g., kids versus elderly).

3.4.4.3 Semiotics in the context of new product development and functional foods

Arning (2016) in his discussion of commercial semiotics applied to brands and marketing suggests various ways that semiotics can be used: advertisement proposition development; product design; brand creation; design innovation; brand revamp; logo design; packaging audit; and design inspiration. Semiotics can be used in packaging design of functional foods to position in the marketplace in relation to competitors. The methodology can be used to evaluate a product category for colours, designs, logos, and then consumers can revaluate newly developed packaging. In 2021, the famous Czech beer brand Pilsner Urquell revealed new packaging for their iconic 300 mL and 500 mL pilsners (Asahi International, 2021). The new bottle showed several distinctive points, and it replaced a retro-inspired brown bottle design launched in 2015. The new bottle featured elongated shoulders, which gave the entire bottle a more modern and dynamic look. For the first time, the brand's symbol was embossed in the cork, not printed, which gave it a premium feel. The key driver for the label redesign was to reduce waste and support sustainability: the firm replaced the golden foil and the plastic stickers with paper materials, making the entire bottle 100% recyclable. The changes put sustainability at the heart of the Pilsner Urquell brand. In the promotional campaign, Pilsner Urquell used sustainability to gain acceptance and approval from consumers. In addition, they gave the "brewery gates", "wax seal", and "city shield" on the bottle increased prominence in the redesign, to really highlight Czech craft, heritage, and provenance. Similar examples could inspire marketers to adjust the functional food packaging to current trends and consumer needs, with particular emphasis on convenience.

3.4.4.4 Selected business and market issues that can be addressed through semiotics

- What does current packaging reveal about the brand and values?
- What colours, logos, signs, and symbols on the packaging create meaning for target consumers?
- Do the colours, logos, signs, and symbols on the packaging reflect the desired positioning in the marketplace?
- For new functional foods, can we effectively communicate product differences?
- What functional claims are important for the target consumers and how can we incorporate them into the packaging?
- How do target consumers define convenient packaging?

3.4.4.5 Selected steps in conducting a semiotics study for functional foods

1. Research the current trends on functional foods related to how consumers use these and similar products.
2. Where does the functional food fit in the NPD process (e.g., idea generation or testing and validation)?
3. Define the problem that needs to be addressed.

4. Conduct focus groups and consumer interviews to get information on functional foods, brands, packaging, and logos.
5. Define the features of the functional foods that are of interest to explore (e.g., pack design, brand, and logos).
6. Conduct a semiotic study to classify information attributes (e.g., brand, pack size, colour) with common meanings and electronically collect the most prominent products in the category you are studying. Interpret the signs and encoded meanings.
7. Clearly define the target market and recruit consumers to interpret visual stimuli based on the focus groups, interviews, and the semiotic sort.
8. Conclude the study and analyse your data and notes.
9. Report on the key findings and answer the research question(s).

3.5 Conclusions

This chapter outlined the importance of a market-oriented approach to developing new functional foods, through integrating consumer information into all stages of the NPD process to avoid marketing myopia within an organisation. Four methodologies were introduced that can be used to gather consumer insights when developing new functional foods and specific examples illustrated their different uses. Each methodology has its advantages and challenges, and their use should be considered according to the nature of the required information, available resources, and the type of product being developed and its stage on the NPD process, for example, is it at the idea generation or launch stages. The next chapter continues with additional market-oriented methodologies for driving functional food development within firms.

References

Arning, C., 2020. Chapter 3: What can semiotics contribute to packging design? In: Maasik, S., Solomon, J. (Eds.), Signs of Life in the USA: Readings on Pop Culture for Writers. Bedford/St. Martin's, Boston, MA/New York, NY.

Arning, C., 2016. Becoming a commercial semiotician. Semiotica 2016 (213), 345–363. https://doi.org/10.1515/sem-2015-0155.

Asahi International, 2021. The same original Pilsner Urquell with new 100% recyclable paper labels. https://www.asahiinternational.com/stories/responsibility/the-same-original-pilsner-urquell-with-new-100-recyclable-paper-labels/# (accessed May 15, 2021).

Belzile, J.A., Öberg, G., 2012. Where to begin? Grappling with how to use participant interaction in focus group design. Qualitative Res. 12 (4), 459–472. https://doi.org/10.1177/1468794111433089.

Bignell, J., 2002. Media Semiotics: An Introduction. Manchester University Press, Manchester, United Kingdom.

Bogue, J., Troy, A-J., 2016. Section I: Market Trends, Regulations, Chemistry, and Health Aspects. Functional beverages: market trends and market-oriented new product design. In: Shahidi, F., Alasalvar, C. (Eds.), Handbook of Functional Beverages and Human Health. Taylor and Francis CRC Press, New York, NY, pp. 3–16.

Braun, V., Clarke, V., 2006. Using thematic analysis in psychology. Qualitative Res. Psychol. 3 (2), 77–101. https://doi.org/10.1191/1478088706qp063oa.

Brown, C.A., Revette, A.C., de Ferranti, S.D., Fontenot, H.B., Gooding, H.C., 2021. Conducting web-based focus groups with adolescents and young adults. Int. J. Qualitative Methods 20, 1–8. https://doi.org/10.1177/1609406921996872.

Caliandro, A., 2018. Digital methods for ethnography: analytical concepts for ethnographers exploring social media environments. J. Contemporary Ethnography 47 (5), 551–578. https://doi.org/10.1177/0891241617702960.

Chesbrough, H., 2020. Open Innovation Results: Going Beyond the Hype and Getting Down to Business. Oxford University Press, Oxford, United Kingdom.

Colom, A., 2021. Using WhatsApp for focus group discussions: ecological validity, inclusion and deliberation. Qualitative Res., 1–16 10.1177/1468794120986074.

Cong, L., Bremer, P., Mirosa, M., 2019. Chinese consumers' perceptions of functional foods: a netnography study of foods that help the immune system recover from air pollution. J. Food Products Market. 25 (6), 628–646. https://doi.org/10.1080/10454446.2019.1 626316.

Conroy, D.M., Gan, C., Errmann, A., Young, J., 2021. Fortifying wellbeing: How Chinese consumers and doctors navigate the role of functional foods. Appetite 164, 105296. https://doi.org/10.1016/j.appet.2021.105296.

Cooper, R.G., 2006. The seven principles of the latest stage-gate® method add up to a streamlined, new product idea-to-launch process. http://www.five-is.com/wp-content/uploads/2013/12/Cooper_2006_Formula_for_Success.pdf (accessed March 19, 2021).

Estey, T., 2019. *The art and science of ethnographic marketing research.* (Online, www.medium. com, February 3, 2019). https://medium.com/@tasha.estey/the-art-science-of-ethnographic-marketing-research-49e703234c00 (accessed June 20, 2021).

Farnsworth, J., Boon, B., 2010. Analysing group dynamics within the focus group. Qualitative Res. 10 (5), 605–624. https://doi.org/10.1177/1468794110375223.

Garcia Martinez, M., 2017. Inspiring crowdsourcing communities to create novel solutions: competition design and the mediating role of trust. Technological Forecasting Social Change 117, 296–304. https://doi.org/10.1016/j.techfore.2016.11.015.

Gobo, G., Cellini, E., 2021. Chapter 7: Ethnographic approaches: types, trends and themes. In: Silverman, D. (Ed.), Qualitative Research. SAGE Publications Ltd., London, United Kingdom, pp. 109–127.

Goffin, K., Lemke, F., Koners, U., 2010. Identifying Hidden Needs: Creating Breakthrough Products. Palgrave Macmillan, Hampshire, United Kingdom/New York, NY.

Halkier, B., 2010. Focus groups as social enactments: integrating interaction and content in the analysis of focus group data. Qualitative Res. 10 (1), 71–89. https://doi. org/10.1177/1468794109348683.

Halliday, M., Mill, D., Johnson, J., Lee, K., 2021. Let's talk virtual! Online focus group facilitation for the modern researcher. Res. Social Adm. Pharm. 17 (12), 2145–2150. https://doi.org/10.1016/j.sapharm.2021.02.003.

Harmsen, H., 1994. Tendencies in product development in danish food companies-report of a qualitative analysis, MAPP Working Paper No. 17. https://pure.au.dk/ws/files/32299736/wp17.pdf (accessed April 21, 2021).

Harmsen, H., Grunert, K.G., Declerck, F., 2000. Why did we make that cheese? An empirically based framework for understanding what drives innovation activity. R & D Manag. 30 (2), 151–166. https://doi.org/10.1111/1467-9310.00165.

Hennink, M.M., 2014. Focus Group Discussions: Understanding Qualitative Research. Oxford University Press, New York, NY.

Hine, C., 2020. Ethnography for the Internet: Embedded, Embodied and Everyday. Routledge, Oxon, United Kingdom/New York, NY.

Kozinets, R.V., 2021. Netnography today: a call to evolve, embrace, energize, and electrify. In: Kozinets, R.V., Gambetti, R. (Eds.), Netnography Unlimited: Understanding Technoculture Using Qualitative Social Media Research. Routledge, Oxon, United Kingdom/New York, NY, pp. 3–23.

Kozinets, R.V., 2015. Netnography: Redefined. SAGE Publications Inc., Thousand Oaks, CA.

Kozinets, R.V., 2010. Netnography: Doing Ethnographic Research Online. SAGE Publications Inc., Thousand Oaks, CA.

Krueger, R.A., Casey, M.A., 2015. Focus Groups: A Practical Guide for Applied Research. SAGE Publications Inc., Thousand Oaks, CA.

Lamphere, L., 2018. The transformation of ethnography: from Malinowski's tent to the practice of collaborative/activist anthropology. Hum. Organ. 77 (1), 64–76. https://doi. org/10.17730/1938-3525.77.1.64.

Lewis, C., Mehmet, M., 2021. An autoethnographic exploration of rural travel with a food intolerance. J. Hospitality Tourism Manag. 47, 289–293. https://doi.org/10.1016/j. jhtm.2021.02.011.

Liamputtong, P., 2011. Chapter 1: Focus Group Methodology: Introduction and History. Focus Group Methodology: Principles and Practice. SAGE Publications Inc., Thousand Oaks, CA., pp. 1–15. https://dx.doi.org/10.4135/9781473957657.

Malinowski, B., 1922. Argonauts of the Western Pacific: An Account of Native Enterprise and Adventure in the Archipelagoes of Melanesian new Guinea. Routledge, London, United Kingdom.

Mellentin, J., 2014. Failures in Functional Foods and Beverages: 12 Reasons Brands Fail and 10 Rules for Success. New Nutrition Business, London, United Kingdom.

Merton, R.K., Fiske, M., Kendall, P.L., 1956. The Focused Interview. The Free Press, New York, NJ.

Moisander, J., Närvänen, E., Valtonen, A., 2020. Chapter 15: Interpretive marketing research: using ethnography in strategic market development. In: Visconti, L., Peñaloza, L., Toulouse, N. (Eds.), Marketing Management: A Cultural Perspective. Routledge, Oxon, United Kingdom/New York, NY, pp. 237–251. https://doi. org/10.4324/9780203710807.

Narver, J.C., Slater, S.T., 1990. The effect of a market orientation on business profitability. J. Market. 54 (4), 20–35. https://doi.org/10.2307/1251757.

Ofstehage, A., 2021. Chapter 16: Soylent: the cultural politics of functional and tasteless food. In: AyoraDiaz, S.I. (Ed.), The Cultural Politics of Food, Taste, and Identity A Global Perspective. Bloomsbury Academic, London, United Kingdom, pp. 242–253. http:// dx.doi.org/10.5040/9781350162754.0024.

Petty, J.N., Thomson, O.P., Stew, G., 2012. Ready for a paradigm shift? Part 2: Introducing qualitative research methodologies and methods. Man. Ther. 17, 378–384. https://doi. org/10.1016/j.math.2012.03.004.

Pink, S., Horst, H., Postill, J., Hjorth, L., Lewis, T., Tacchi, J., 2015. Digital Ethnography: Principles and Practice. SAGE Publications Ltd., London, United Kingdom.

Podnar, K., Balmer, J.M.T., 2021. Quo Vadis Corporate Marketing? J. Business Res. 134, 642–646. https://doi.org/10.1016/j.jbusres.2021.06.015.

Pountney, L., Marić, T., 2021. Introducing Anthropology: What Makes Us Human? Polity Press, Cambridge, United Kingdom.

Princeton, 2021. What is Ethnography? The Trustees of Princeton University, Princeton, NJ. https://anthropology.princeton.edu/undergraduate/ethnographic-studies/what-ethnography (Accessed April 6, 2021).

Reeves, S., Kuper, A., Hodges, B.D., 2008. Qualitative research methodologies: ethnography. British Med. J. 337, a1020. https://doi.org/10.1136/bmj.a1020.

Reid, D.J., Reid, F.J.M., 2005. Online focus groups: an in-depth comparison of computer-mediated and conventional focus group discussions. Int. J. Market Res. 47 (2), 131–162. https://doi.org/10.1177/147078530504700204.

Relich, M., 2021. Chapter 1: Product development: state of the art and challenges. Decision Support for Product Development: Using Computational Intelligence for information Acquisition in Enterprise Databases. Springer Nature, Cham, Switzerland, pp. 1–26. https://doi.org/10.1007/978-3-030-43897-5_1#DOI.

Richard, B., Sivo, S.A., Orlowski, M., Ford, R.C., Murphy, J., Boote, D.N., Witta, E.L., 2020. Qualitative research via focus groups: will going online affect the diversity of your findings? Cornel Hospitality Quart. 62 (1), 32–45. https://doi.org/10.1177/1938965520967769.

Savin-Baden, M., Howell Major, C., 2013. Qualitative Research: The essential guide to theory and practice. Routledge, London, United Kingdom/New York, NY.

Sorenson, D., Bogue, J., 2009. Chapter 17: Consumer-oriented development of functional beverages. In: Paquin, P. (Ed.), Functional and Speciality Beverage Technology. Woodhead Publishing, Elsevier, Cambridge, United Kingdom, pp. 421–450. https://doi.org/10.1533/9781845695569.4.421.

Soylent, 2021. Company's website. https://soylent.com/(accessed June 12, 2021).

Taylor, B.C., 2017. Ethnography. In: Scott, C.R., Lewis, L. (Eds.), The International Encyclopedia of Organizational Communication. Wiley-Blackwell, West Sussex, United Kingdom. https://doi.org/10.1002/9781118955567.wbieoc076.

United Nations, 2020. *World Population Ageing 2020: Highlights.* https://www.un.org/development/desa/pd/sites/www.un.org.development.desa.pd/files/undesa_pd-2020_world_population_ageing_highlights.pdf (accessed June 26, 2021).

van Trijp, C.M., van Kleef, E., 2008. Newness, value and new product performance. Trends Food Sci. Technol. 19 (11), 562–573. https://doi.org/10.1016/j.tifs.2008.03.004.

Valentin, D., Gómez-Corona, C., 2018. Chapter 5: Using ethnography in consumer research. In: Ares, G., Varela, P. (Eds.), Methods in Consumer Research: New Approaches to Classic Methods, Volume 1. Woodhead Publishing Series in Food Science, Technology and Nutrition. Elsevier, Cambridge, United Kingdom, pp. 103–123. https://doi.org/10.1016/B978-0-08-102089-0.00005-4.

Vindrola-Padros, C., 2021. Rapid Ethnographies: A Practical Guide. Cambridge University Press, Cambridge, United Kingdom.

Wilkinson, S., 2020. Chapter 6: Analysing focus group data. In: Silverman, D. (Ed.), Qualitative Research. SAGE Publications Ltd., London, pp. 87–104.

Wunsch, N.-G. (2020). *Global functional food market revenue 2013 and 2022.* https://www.statista.com/statistics/252803/global-functional-food-sales/(accessed June 13, 2021).

CHAPTER 4

Market-oriented methodologies that integrate the consumer into the functional foods new product development process: Part 2 advanced approaches

Lana Repar, Joe Bogue
Department of Food Business and Development, Cork University Business School, University College Cork, Ireland

4.1 Introduction

In the previous chapter, the importance of a market-oriented approach to new product development (NPD), for developing new products, or modifying existing products, was seen as key to success in competitive and ever-evolving consumer markets. This chapter presents three advanced market-oriented methodologies that integrate consumer insights into the process for developing new functional foods. The methodologies covered in this chapter include sensory analysis, conjoint analysis, and new technologies that can be used to generate market-oriented consumer insights.

4.2 Sensory analysis

4.2.1 History and recent developments

Most methodologies for exploring consumer insights test either the product concept, or consumers' perceptions, and how the product is being used. Sensory analysis is the only method that tests the sensory appeal of foods, and this information is critical for the development of successful functional foods. This methodology investigates human senses in relation to food products, such as taste, texture, appearance, and smell. During the 1940s and 1950s, the foundations for sensory analysis were developed by the US Army Quartermaster Food and Container Institute, which supported research in food acceptance for the armed forces (Peryam et al., 1954). Rose Marie Pangborn was one of the pioneers in the field of sensory analysis of food attributes, publishing over 180 scientific articles. The initial efforts to understand which foods were more, or less preferred, were nearly forgotten during the 1960s and early 1970s, as the focus shifted to feeding the growing population, rather than determining whether the sensory properties of foods were acceptable to the targeted groups (Stone and Sidel, 2004).

Sensory analysis has an important role to play in relation to consumer acceptance of novel foods: protein-based foods made from insects, part meat and part plant hybrid foods, plant-based foods, and the development of new fish products made from sustainable species. In addition, recent developments in this methodology explore the link between sensory studies and nutrition in relation to calorific intake. For example, McCrickerd and Forde (2016) examined how certain sensory characteristics can be used to promote better energy intake control. They suggest that sensory signals generated by food could be used in a way that might promote better food choices in consumers and energy intake regulation, by influencing how much they eat, and how they eat it, beyond how much food is liked. Rapid sensory methods with trained panels are the future of consumer sensory analysis as they will achieve the advantages of speed and reliability, and this will be enhanced by technology enabling real-time testing using tablets, mobile phones, and social media fora (Kemp et al., 2018). Furthermore, if we combine sensory and marketing research together into sensory marketing, we can deal with measurements of what fascinates the consumer through the senses (Poretta, 2021).

4.2.2 Sensory analysis procedure, advantages, and challenges

Sensory analysis can be performed using both experts and regular consumers. Trained experts provide qualitative descriptions and develop the vocabulary for specific food and beverage categories. Regular or "naïve" consumers are often presented with several prototypes and a hedonic scale to capture their opinions regarding preferences for taste, texture, and smell of specific foods under investigation. Ranking these items on a hedonic scale allows the identification of different consumer clusters or segments and ultimately increases the chances of success for a new food product. The benefits of sensory analysis are numerous: it helps to direct product development at an intrinsic level; identifies consumer clusters through sensory segmentation; and assists in marketing for product positioning and communication of product attributes targeted at specific consumer segments. However, undertaking sensory analysis requires prior experience and knowledge, having health and safety procedures in place, and can be time-consuming. The common types of sensory analysis methods for functional food product development are outlined in Table 4.1.

Sensory and market analysis are inextricably linked, with sensory analysis and marketing identifying the intrinsic and extrinsic attributes of food products respectively. One of the first steps at the early stages of the NPD process is for the entrepreneur or product developer to conduct sensory analysis on identified competitors in the marketplace. This reveals the sensory profiles of competitors' products and identifies opportunities to develop products with different sensory profiles in terms of taste, texture, appearance, and smell. Through conducting hedonic sensory evaluation, we can identify which of the competitor's products are most liked by consumers and then group those consumers into segments linked to their socio-economic profiles. Furthermore, we can then get the trained expert sensory panelists to identify the key sensory attributes of the most popular products and link these to the identified segments. Looking at factors for developing successful functional foods, Mellentin (2009) identified taste of a functional food as one of the basic factors to get right, which is highly relevant to the target market.

4.2.3 Sensory analysis in the context of the new product development and functional foods

Sensory analysis is important at the end of the development process, at the testing and validation phase, and for quality purposes. It can also be used at the early design stage to profile competitor products and identify market opportunities. For functional foods, this method can be used at a critical moment where consumers provide their subjective judgements of the product. Taste, texture, and smell play a significant role in consumers' choices as they often dictate food choices, consumers' preferences, and calorific intake. Sensory analysis of functional foods is especially relevant for those foods with modified ingredients, such as gluten-free and dairy-free. By removing certain ingredients, a food product generally changes in terms of its intrinsic characteristics. Sensory analysis can reveal to what extent consumers are willing to accept changes in taste and texture profiles.

Table 4.1 Common types of sensory analysis methods for functional foods.

No.	Type	Procedure	Relevance for functional foods
	Difference or Discrimination Tests (usually 25–40 assessors)	**Assessors, sometimes trained, compare various samples to determine whether they are the same or different. They might provide a score or a grade to the sample, or comment on why they believe the samples are different**	
1.	A–Not A	Assessors are given at least two samples from which at least one of them is sample "A" and at least one of them is a test sample (Not A). They determine whether the sample they are evaluating is sample "A" or "Not A." Some variations include monadic, paired, replicated monadic, replicated mixed, and replicated paired method	Quality control, product sorting or screening, panel training, and NPD directed at children and the elderly as a target market
2.	Multiple-samples ranking test	Assessors rank a given set of samples regarding the increasing or decreasing preference or sensory attribute intensity	
3.	Paired comparison	Assessors determine which of the two samples is stronger or more intense in a specific attribute of interest (e.g., bitter or sweeter).	
4.	Duo–trio	Assessors determine which of the two given samples is the closest to a third sample identified as a reference	
5.	Triangle test	Assessors are given three samples. They need to determine which two samples are the same, or which sample is most different from the two other samples	
6.	Tetrad test	Assessors are given four samples, two samples of one product and two samples of another product. They group the samples into two groups according to their similarity—the samples in each group are more similar to each other than the other two samples	

No.	Type	Procedure	Relevance for functional foods
Affective or Hedonic Tests (usually 75–150 assessors)		**Usually untrained (naïve) assessors rate their liking or acceptance of appearance, aroma, flavour and texture of the samples, and express their overall impression**	
1.	Sensory acceptance test	Assessors are regular consumers of a product. They assess overall acceptance and preferences or liking of specific attributes on a nine-point hedonic scale	Product development, nutritional optimisation and validation, identification of different consumer segments based on different attributes (e.g., flavours or colours), and information on consumer acceptance of functional foods
2.	Consumer acceptance test	A sensory acceptance test on a large scale	
3.	Preference tests	Assessors reveal which product(s) they prefer over the others. The ranking is sometimes used	
4.	Flash profiling	Assessors generate their own free-choice attributes to describe the samples and can see other assessors' attributes to add or substitute attributes in their list. Assessors then rank the samples according to their intensity for each developed attribute on an ordinal scale from "lower" to "higher"	

(Continued)

Table 4.1 Cont'd

No.	Type	Procedure	Relevance for functional foods
	Descriptive Tests (usually 10–12 assessors)	**Trained assessors quantitatively measure the sensory attributes of appearance, aroma, flavour, texture, taste, and aftertaste. The terminology is descriptive and nonhedonic**	
1.	Flavour profile method (FPM)	Through a group discussion, consensus technique, vocabulary development, and rating sessions, the assessors characterize all the flavour components and their intensities in a food product	Throughout the product life-cycle: market mapping, product development, value optimisation, packaging, protection of signature sensory characteristics that form a brand mix, and quality control
2.	Texture profile method (TPM)	Assessors determine the rheological and tactile characteristics of a food product from first bite through mastication, using a set of force-related and shape-related texture attribute scales	
3.	Quantitative descriptive analysis (QDA)	Trained assessors assess perceived intensity and quality of samples. The samples might be presented in a sequential monadic way where all the attributes for each sample are assessed, or all samples are assessed on each attribute. Instead of reaching a consensus via discussion, the data are usually averaged across all the assessors and statistical analyses are used	
4.	Spectrum Method	Intensively trained assessors use a strict technical sensory vocabulary and pre learned intensity scales to score perceived intensities of the attributes from given samples	
5.	Free choice profiling (FCP)	Assessors (trained, or untrained) develop their own descriptive terms instead of using a common vocabulary, and then rate the samples accordingly	

Source: Adapted based on Bi and Ennis (1999), Carabante and Prinyawiwatkul (2018), Dehlholm et al. (2012), Kemp et al. (2018), Lawless and Heymann (2010), O'Sullivan (2017), Piggott et al. (1998), and Punter (2018).

4.2.4 Selected business and market issues that can be addressed through sensory analysis

- What sensory profile does the target market prefer?
- Do consumers accept the sensory profile of a new product/ingredient?
- How do the functional food products compare on a sensory basis with those of the competitors?
- Can we segment the market on a sensory basis?
- Can the sensory profile of the functional foods be the unique selling point?
- Can we reformulate the functional food product with healthier/cheaper ingredients?

Box 4.1   Whatever makes sense-different facets of sensory analysis

Sensory analysis reveals information relevant for understanding consumer preferences when developing new functional foods. There are various ways to undertake sensory analysis, depending on the novelty of the product, consumers' familiarity with an ingredient or acceptance of the sensory profile. A sensory study can emphasise the testing of the scientific composition of a new functional food, or it could focus more on consumer preferences. For example, Cais-Sokolińska and Walkowiak-Tomczak (2021) performed a set of scientific analyses (compositional and physicochemical analysis; bioactive compounds and antioxidant capacity; estimation of hypoglycemic ability; and in vitro gastrointestinal digestion simulation) for their yogurt with restructured elderberry juice before undertaking consumer sensory analysis. Similarly, De Farias Silva et al. (2021) began their study with scientific analysis of fruit pulp and rice protein agglomerated with collagen (agglomeration process of concentrated rice protein powder; characterization of raw and agglomerated rice protein; and colour and viscosity analysis) and followed up with consumer sensory analysis. In contrast, Michell et al. (2021) structured their study by first exploring consumer sensory perceptions and acceptability of microgreens, and then used a questionnaire and principal component analysis to further understand factors influencing acceptability, sensory perceptions, and consumers' intent to purchase microgreens. Crucean et al. (2019) took a different approach and introduced a reduced salt bread enriched with vitamin B4 to French consumers. They undertook a sensory test at the beginning, then deepened their understanding of consumers' acceptance of the product and the optimal target market, through a series of focus groups.

The four studies above used different types of sensory analysis, as follows. For their descriptive sensory analysis, Cais-Sokolińska and Walkowiak-Tomczak (2021) used a profiling method with a panel of 13 members, who were trained for approximately 36 h and identified descriptors by evaluating yogurt samples on 9-cm unstructured line scales (low-high). Additionally, the authors used 107 consumers in visual sensory tests to rate likeness on a 9-point hedonic scale (like extremely-dislike extremely), as well as in consumer penalty analysis where they rated aroma, flavour, colour, and texture on a 5-point just-about-right (JAR) scale (1 = not enough, 3 = ideal, 5 = too much). De Farias Silva et al. (2021) recruited between 25 and 30 consumers of fruits and fruit pulps to rate the flavour, aroma, colour, smell, and appearance of different juices on a 9-point hedonic scale (dislike extremely-like extremely). Michell et al. (2020) used a convenient sample of 99 consumers, who rated six different microgreens species and performed sensory perception evaluation on a nine-category horizontal line scale (none-strongest imaginable), and acceptance evaluation of appearance, texture, and flavour on a 9-point hedonic scale (highly unacceptable-highly acceptable). Crucean et al. (2019) performed a sensory ranking test, where 32 assessors ranked bread samples from the lowest (rank 1) to the highest salty taste (rank 5). In addition, 40 assessors were used in a triangle test where they were simultaneously given three bread samples (two identical and one different) and had to identify the different samples.

Using sensory analysis, and complementing it with quantitative or qualitative methods, allows full integration of consumers into the new functional food development process. In the four studies above, sensory analysis was employed to: (1) explore consumers' acceptance and determine the optimal sensory properties of functional foods; (2) optimise the formulation of new functional foods; (3) understand consumers' preferences for new functional foods and identify target markets; (4) pinpoint the information and educational aspects that consumers require about new functional foods; and (5) take a deep dive into whether functional foods evoke any reflections on cultural and symbolic representations of food, and explore the intent to purchase new functional foods.

Case study based on Cais-Sokolińska and Walkowiak-Tomczak (2021), Crucean et al. (2019), De Farias Silva et al. (2021), and Michell et al. (2020).

4.2.5 Selected steps in conducting sensory analysis for functional foods

1. Research the current trends on functional foods related to consumer sensory preferences.
2. Where does the functional food fit in the NPD process (e.g., idea generation or testing and validation)?
3. Define the problem that needs to be addressed.
4. Decide on the type of sensory analysis that is the most appropriate, as well as the participants (e.g., naïve or expert panel). Consider the type of analysis (e.g., qualitative vs quantitative) that will be required for the study.
5. Develop a detailed protocol and secure an appropriate conditions and location for the sensory analysis (e.g., temperature–controlled room, appropriate lighting, computer software, etc.).

6. Prepare the required samples.
7. Recruit and train the participants (depending on their role and previous expertise).
8. Conduct sensory analysis and record data.
9. Depending on the collected data, use analytical methods for qualitative/quantitative data.
10. Report on the key findings and answer the research question(s).

4.3 Conjoint analysis

4.3.1 History and recent developments

Conjoint analysis is a powerful predictive marketing tool that can be used to examine consumer preferences for a range of product attributes and, ultimately, a complete product. It emanated from work in the 1960s by mathematical psychologists and statisticians and was developed further for use in business and marketing by Green and Rao (1971) through their seminal work *Conjoint Measurement for Quantifying Judgmental Data*. This method has been widely used for NPD purposes due to its advantages when it comes to singling out and comparing features or attributes that constitute a product. Conjoint analysis relies on developments in software and statistical analysis, and its progress will be underpinned by the advances in these two areas. Several software are currently available for performing this methodology, such as *SPSS, Qualtrics, Conjointly, Sawtooth Software*, and *1000 minds*. Future conjoint analyses are likely to utilise the advantages of augmented reality simulations, to create real-life purchasing situations and gather more accurate data (Petit et al., 2021).

Before delving into conjoint analysis, it is worth mentioning the consumer survey as a methodology that has been used extensively in market research. Compared to conjoint analysis, a consumer survey is less complex in the design process, but often uses sophisticated statistics and econometric tests in the analysis stage, and this is where its strength lies. A consumer survey is a form of a questionnaire and consists of a set of questions, usually grouped into meaningful sections, which can take different forms: open-ended (e.g., precise number or shorter narrative) or close-ended type of questions, for example, single choice, multiple-choice, ranking on a Likert scale or numerical scale, rating and agreement/disagreement with a statement. A consumer survey can address many different business and marketing issues and can be distributed to a large number of participants in a relatively short period of time. Nowadays, various software, such as

Google Forms, Office 365 Forms, Survey Monkey, LimeSurvey, and *Qualtrics* support the creation, distribution, and analysis of data collected for a consumer survey. A key to an effective functional foods consumer survey is the selection of suitable questions and the type of required responses, that will later serve as variables for different analytical tests. In addition, the effective recruitment of an appropriate sample is important, which can be achieved through filter questions at the start of the survey.

Results from consumer surveys are highly valuable for the development of functional foods. For example, Nan et al. (2017) examined predictors of American consumers' preferences for fortified foods using a sample of 6728 respondents. Using OLS multiple regression analysis, this study showed that females, those that were more educated and health-conscious had greater preferences for fortified foods. In another study, Nystrand and Olsen (2020) explored attitudes and intentions for consumption of functional foods among 810 Norwegian consumers. Through structural equation modelling, the results highlighted that utilitarian eating values outperformed hedonic eating values in terms of consumers' attitudes towards functional foods consumption, and the authors importantly suggested that food firms need to improve the hedonic value of functional foods to make them more commercially successful. In China, Huang et al. (2020) investigated the effects of the "carrier," "benefit," and "trust in information channel" on the purchase of functional foods in the case of 1114 respondents. Data were analysed using repeated and one-way ANOVA, two-step clustering analysis, and principal components analysis, and revealed that: (1) "the carrier" was a more important factor than "benefits" for perceived attractiveness and purchase intention; (2) the most favoured benefits were "improving (the) body's natural defence system"; and (3) "the perceived trust in friends" recommendation' scored the highest. The value of consumer surveys, for novel functional food development, is also reflected in Torri et al. (2020) who examined the attitudes of 1445 Italian consumers towards consuming jellyfish, a source of bioactive compounds. Principal component analysis, two-way ANOVA, hierarchical multiple linear regression and correspondence analysis revealed that jellyfish is most likely to be accepted by young people with high education levels, or students familiar with the marine environment and frequent travellers. The application of consumer surveys in determining the acceptance of novel functional foods has the potential to identify the early adopters, but also detect potential challenges, such as neophobia and disgust as pointed out by Torri et al. (2020), and eliminate them before introducing a new product to the market.

4.3.2 Selected business and market issues that can be addressed through a consumer survey

- What are consumers' habits, attitudes, perceptions, and preferences for functional foods?
- What are the key drivers for functional food consumption/nonconsumption?
- What is the socio-demographic profile of the potential target market?
- What are determinants of functional food consumption and what consumer profile is more likely to consume functional foods?

4.3.3 Conjoint procedure, advantages, and challenges

A significant advantage of conjoint analysis is its ability to answer various *what if* questions using market simulators; these simulators are based on the results of an analysis of conjoint data collected on hypothetical and real choice alternatives (Rao, 2014). There are several types of conjoint analyses and they are all based on a questionnaire, either hard copy or online, where respondents choose from a set of hypothetical options on the principle of trade-offs. The way in which those trade-offs are formatted varies from one conjoint type to another (see Table 4.2). Depending on the type, respondents might assess a full profile or several attributes, and they either rate the concepts or choose among two to three bundles. The output of a conjoint analysis is usually a full product profile, or a set of key attribute levels, that consumers are likely to choose in the retail marketplace. It is a very useful methodology to give guidance to product developers, prior to going into the product development laboratory to start developing product prototypes.

Once hypothetical products have been created, a conjoint analysis questionnaire is designed. Depending on the type of conjoint analysis, the questionnaire might contain either a hedonic scale for consumers to rank each hypothetical product (rank-based) or selection between two or three hypothetical product options (choice-based). In addition, the conjoint analysis questionnaire will also contain socio-demographic questions, as this will serve as a basis for identifying consumer clusters. The outputs from the conjoint analysis will reveal the attribute level utilities, or how much importance each attribute level has upon the overall product preference, as well as different consumer clusters and their socio-demographic characteristics. Information from the conjoint analysis assists in combining product attribute levels in a way that is attractive to an identified consumer cluster, which increases the chances of market success.

Table 4.2 Types and characteristics of conjoint analysis for functional foods.

No.	Type	Procedure	Relevance for functional foods
Rating-based method		**Participants rank or rate a series of full-profile products, one product at a time** (usually up to 8 attributes and 5 attribute levels)	Estimating the impact of each attribute level on overall product prefer-
1.	Traditional (CA) or full-profile	Respondents are presented with full-profiles of hypothetical products, including the entire set of attributes. Respondents rate full-profiles on a Likert scale according to their preferences	ence; making decisions on product characteristics, packaging, branding, and price for a new functional food product based on
Choice-Based Methods		**Participants are shown a set of full-profile products and they select which one they would purchase** (usually lots of attributes and up to 5 attribute levels)	different attributes and attribute levels
1.	Choice-based (CBCA) or discrete choice	Respondents are presented with 2–3 bundles from which they need to select the most preferred one	
2.	Adaptive choice-based (ACDCA)	Respondents are presented with multiple bundles to choose from, and as they progress, the bundles are becoming more relevant to them, which is based on their previous responses	
3.	Self-explicated	Uses a bottom-up approach. Respondents are first shown the attributes and their levels and asked to identify any of the levels that is so unat-tractive that any choice with such attribute level would be rejected. Second, respondents rate their best and worst attribute level within each attribute. Then they rate the remaining levels for the same attri-butes on a scale from 0 to 10. Furthermore, the respondents are asked to rate the most valuable upgrade across all the attributes to determine how important attributes are, relative to each other. Finally, the respon-dents allocate 100 points among the top-level attributes	

No.	Type	Procedure	Relevance for functional foods
4.	Menu-based (MBCA)	Respondents are introduced to all of the attributes, and attribute levels used in the study, and asked to build their own packages in accordance with their preferences. The price is used as a constraint and it is updated based on the options selected by the respondents	
5.	Perceptual choice	An extension of the choice-based type. It contains a question after each discrete choice task on why the respondents selected a particular bundle. The answer options represent perceptual items tied to each bundle	
6.	Volumetric	Similar to the choice-based type, but the respondents state how many units of each offered bundle they would purchase	

Source: Adapted based on Lutz (2021), Orme (2010), Rao (2014), and Srinivasan and Park (1997).

Although it is one of the most used quantitative methods in consumer research and NPD, difficulty with conjoint analysis is that it assumes consumers will behave in the same way when they are actually purchasing their products. However, it disregards the fact that often brands and packaging play a significant role for consumers during the purchase situation. Hence, instead of using typical text-based questions, newer research by Velázquez et al. (2021) used visual representation of the product to simulate the actual purchase scenario. Another challenge with conjoint analysis is respondent fatigue that might occur if the study design requires respondents to select among numerous hypothetical products, one after another. This can decrease respondents' attention to detail and motivation to complete the conjoint questionnaire, and impact the reliability of the results.

4.3.4 Conjoint in the context of new product development and functional foods

Conjoint analysis is suitable in the concept generation stages of NPD. It first requires a set of product attributes and attribute levels that will be explored. The attributes represent the relevant aspects of a product identified by consumers, while the attribute levels reflect options for each attribute that could be potentially incorporated in a product design. One of the approaches to conjoint analysis is to use focus group discussions as a scoping study to ascertain relevant attributes for functional foods, and subsequently to use expert interviews to frame the attribute levels. Findings from the focus group discussions, coupled with expert interviews, can provide a basis for conjoint analysis and the generation of hypothetical functional foods in the computer software, such as *SPSS*. Relevant attributes of functional foods include brand, carrier, flavour, texture, price per weight, functionality, type of packaging, and label information.

4.3.5 Selected business and market issues that can be addressed through conjoint analysis

- What is the most important attribute driving consumer preferences?
- What are the trade-offs that consumers make among the different attribute levels?
- Can we identify specific products and corresponding consumer clusters or segments?
- Is there a "functionally driven consumer segment," that is, a group of consumers that would pay extra for foods with added ingredients, which have specific health benefits?

Box 4.2   Conjoint analysis and enriched functional foods

Rebouças et al. (2020) used conjoint analysis to understand consumer preferences in their study on the effect and importance of front label attributes on purchase intention for a new functional beverage containing cashew nuts and mango juice. The authors first conducted focus group discussions to assess consumer choice and front label attributes. Four focus group discussions were held with between 5 and 11 participants per group. The criterion for participant selection was regular consumption of soya milk beverages with added fruit juice. From here, a combination of attributes and attribute levels resulted in 18 labels, which were further analysed using conjoint and cluster analysis. The labels were presented via a projector in a meeting room to a total of 126 participants, divided into groups of seven (a total of 18 sessions). Participants assessed the labels using a 9 cm unstructured scale with two anchors at each end, with the left one stating "would definitely not buy it" and the right one stating "would definitely buy it."

At the beginning of the conjoint analysis, all labels to be assessed were shown on a slide, with the intention to simulate the real-life situation in a retail environment and the choice among multiple products when purchasing a functional beverage. In the next step, a slide with a label without the attributes to be assessed was shown, followed by each of the 18 labels and they appeared for 15 seconds, with a 5 second break between them (blank slide). Participants were shown each slide in a monadic way in complete balanced blocks to eliminate the effect of the presentation order and the residual effect of the influence of the previous image. To further fight fatigue, participants were given a 10-min break after assessing the first nine labels. In addition to the conjoint questionnaire, data on demographics, consumption characteristics, and cognitive and attitudinal factors (such as knowledge, acceptance of functional foods, perceived role of food for health, belief in the health benefits, and price perception) were collected. The results from the focus groups and conjoint analysis were compared. The focus groups revealed that the most relevant information was "the illustration," "the nutritional information," and the term "prebiotic." The conjoint analysis confirmed that "the illustration" was the attribute with an important influence on consumers' purchase intention with "the nutritional information" and the term "prebiotic" of lower importance.

A variation of conjoint analysis can be considered in cases where an innovative approach is required with the target market, such as designing functional foods for elderly consumers. Bogue et al. (2017) utilised a user-centred design to optimise the development of new functional foods for the ageing population. The attributes for new functional foods were identified through interviews with key stakeholders and the attribute levels were generated from the relevant literature and in consultation with the marketing and technical NPD team. Thirty-two Irish consumers were then purposively selected and completed a brief demographic questionnaire. During the interactions, the participants were divided into four groups of eight participants. In the first stage, each group was further divided into two subgroups (four participants in each) and, using a designated laptop with preloaded *drag and drop* software, the participants assembled a functional food concept by selecting the desired attribute levels (attributes: "health concerns," "carrier," "packaging," "marketing messages" and "health claims"). In the second stage, the group came together and the two concepts that were designed from the consumer interactions were discussed with a facilitator and focused on: (1) the motives for choosing specific attributes and (2) the appeal of different attribute levels.

Case study based on: Bogue et al. (2017) and Rebouças et al. (2020).

4.3.6 Selected steps in conducting a conjoint analysis study for functional foods

1. Research the current trends on functional foods related to consumer preferences.
2. Where does the functional food fit in the NPD process (e.g., idea generation or testing and validation)?
3. Define the problem that needs to be addressed.
4. Conduct focus groups to identify key consumer issues, motivations to purchase, and key product attributes.
5. Decide on the type of conjoint analysis that is the most appropriate, as well as the profile of participants.
6. Identify the appropriate analysis required to answer your research questions.
7. Select the attributes, and the attribute levels, and run the selected conjoint analysis.
8. Report on the key findings and answer the research question(s).

4.4 New technology developments for consumer insights

New developments in technology that garner consumer insights promise innovative methodologies, which will use vast data, more quickly and with greater precision. For functional food research, the following areas are of interest: (1) big data, (2) mobile applications, and (3) eye tracking. Furthermore, advances in neuroscience facilitate the exploration of consumers' neural functions when making decisions, such as in the study by Contreras-Rodrigues et al. (2020), where the results showed that overweight individuals displayed an increased willingness to pay for functional foods, which might be driven by an activation of the regions of the brain, that direct attention to internal goals. This section will focus on new technology developments for generating consumer insights for developing functional foods.

4.4.1 Big data

Consumers leave digital traces and they do it often throughout the day. Weekly shopping in a local supermarket, or writing a review after purchasing a new product online, creates data. When lots of consumers engage in such activities daily, the amount of data captured is huge. Modern technology enables the automated collection, storage, and analysis of complex and large amounts of data, which makes it possible to turn consumers' digital traces into valuable information on their purchasing behaviour, attitudes, preferences or concerns. Sources of big data relevant for consumers can come from: (1) social data (e.g., websites and social media); (2) machine data (e.g., sensors and smart meters); and transactional data (e.g., online and offline payments) (Blazquez and Domenech, 2018). Big data require sophisticated tools, beyond the traditional data processing applications, such as Excel, and often rely on various algorithms. However, as warned by Lazer et al. (2014) in the case of *Google Flu Trends* (flu tracking system) that has been persistently overestimating flu prevalence, big data are generally not gathered using proven traditional scientific instruments and, therefore, the analysis can sometimes lead to errors.

A debate on how big data could potentially *supplement or even replace traditional survey data in the future* is ongoing (Birkin et al., 2021, p. 4). Nevertheless, big data offer immense opportunities to assist in critical decision-making processes, whether it is a long-term and binding decision, such as the next retail location, or short term, such as what to include in shopper coupons (Aversa et al., 2021). For consumer research, this methodology can generate rich real-time data, relevant for all stages of the consumer decision-making cycle (e.g., *what* people consume, *when* and *with whom*) and it is useful for informing marketing decisions, undertaking marketing campaigns, and translating consumer insights into market advantage (Erevelles et al., 2016; Hofacker et al., 2016).

Matz and Netzer (2017) suggested that using big data allowed real-time "optimisation" of marketing actions and provided a window into consumers' psychological traits. Recent studies have demonstrated some creative use of big data. For example, Park (2019) explored the role of satisfaction on customer intent to reuse airline services by analysing data from 130,000 customers' responses about their online service and in-flight experience. Similarly, Tian et al. (2021) analysed 175,879 text-based online reviews on consumers' dining sentiments to understand the relationship between the sentiment indices and the ratings. In another example, Pantano et al. (2021) reviewed 10,544 consumers' tweets and allowed unsolicited consumer language to reveal what key attributes and concerns matter to consumers to find out what they think about 19 main shopping centres in the UK and implications future retail planning. Furthermore, Hamilton and Lahne (2020) developed a vocabulary of flavour descriptors for whiskey sensory analysis by analysing 6598 online reviews from international whiskies websites, which reduced the time and costs usually required for this protocol.

4.4.2 Selected business and market issues that can be addressed through big data

- What are the new opportunities for our firm's national and global growth?
- What new functional food categories can be developed?
- Who is our typical consumer and what is her/his shopping behaviour?
- What new functional ingredients are appearing on global markets?

4.4.3 Mobile applications

Mobile applications have gained increased popularity in the past decade. With the growth of smartphones, mobile applications have become a staple of everyday life. Nowadays, mobile applications are used across a myriad of different business sectors, from educational and health-related content, to entertainment. Firms that adjust their web content for mobile applications and incorporate seamless mobile purchases can take advantage of this phenomenon. For functional foods, there is a huge opportunity to utilise mobile applications for product innovation and consumer feedback. Firms can develop their mobile applications to increase consumer engagement and gather valuable insights from consumers' activities. For example, *Nestlé* offers several different mobile applications, such as *Nestlé Pure Life* for shopping, *Now@Nestlé* for social networking and *Nestlé Cocina* for recipes. Other uses include mobile applications for research purposes, such as *Indeemo, EthOS, dscout, CrowdLab, Contextmapp* and *Over the Shoulder*, which use AI-powered tools and "imitate" ethnography, to enable participants capture their daily experiences usually via diary, notes, videos, audios, and image uploads. There are also specialized mobile applications, such as *Batterii*, created for innovation, concept testing, and NPD tasks. Different research has shown the role of mobile applications in food research: to identify and analyse the factors influencing the intentions of customers to use mobile applications for ordering food (Samala and Sama, 2018); assessment of nutrition-focused mobile applications influence on consumers' healthy food behaviour and nutrition knowledge (Samoggia and Riedel, 2020); and the Dutch mobile application *FoodProfiler* can track consumer eating habits and be used by industry to tailor their NPD activities (Michail, 2016).

4.4.4 Selected business and market issues that can be addressed through mobile applications

- What are consumers' daily experiences with functional foods? How can we innovate using consumers' artefacts (images, videos, audios) and design successful functional foods that are catering for the needs of our target market?
- What type of consumers shop using mobile applications? How does their journey look like?
- How do consumers use mobile applications to connect with functional food brands?
- How can we increase consumer engagement and loyalty to the brand through a mobile application?
- What kind of mobile applications features are desirable/irrelevant (e.g., information on health, calories or ingredients)?

4.4.5 Eye tracking

The eye-tracking methodology is a technology-supported method of exploring consumer behaviour to understand how they view their shopping surroundings and products. It is often employed to detect which areas of a supermarket, a shelf or product packaging, consumers spend most time looking at during the purchase situation. This information assists marketers in arranging shelf space and designing packaging to increase the effectiveness of shopper experiences. The eye-tracking technology uses heat maps to indicate: (1) where consumers look on the retail shelf space or the packaging (fixation count); (2) how long they spend looking at it (fixation duration); and (3) the order that consumers view it (saccades) (Geisen and Romano Bergstrom, 2017). Huang et al. (2021) used the eye-tracking methodology to explore the colour-flavour non-congruency effect in food labels and suggested that consumers relied on colour cues when they searched for packaging with a certain flavour label. They found that when consumers did not find it through a colour-based search, they switched to a word-based search. In another use of this technology, Puurtinen et al. (2021) discovered that when consumers inspected a salad buffet for 20s and then assembled a self-choice salad, the centrally placed dishes gained relatively more "gaze visits," compared to items places at the corners, though the food colour did not affect visual processing. Interestingly, the authors highlighted that one of the measures, pupil-size, did not function with elderly participants, which reinforced the importance of having a deep understanding of consumer segments. Peng-Li et al. (2021) went one step further and combined the eye-tracking methodology with custom-composed soundtracks to study consumer choices, and demonstrated that "healthy soundtracks" induced more and longer fixations on healthy foods. Through the eye-tracking methodology, firms can gain valuable insights into cues on packaging and product placement that entice different consumer segments to purchase functional foods.

4.4.6 Selected business and market issues that can be addressed through eye tracking

- Which aspects of the packaging are the most important to consumers?
- How long do consumers spend looking at different components of packaging?
- How does location on a shelf impact consumers' purchasing behaviour?
- What information should be emphasised on functional food packaging?
- Where should functional foods be placed (1) in the supermarket and (2) on the shelf?

Box 4.3   Keep an eye on it! Eye tracking and effective food claims

The first impression consumers get about a food product is usually through its packaging. A unique selling point of functional foods is the fact that they provide benefits beyond nutrients and energy. However, during the first purchase, this can often only be captured through a food claim. Steinhauser et al. (2019) used a close-to-realistic purchase situation where 3D packages of orange juice and milk chocolate with accompanying nutrition, health, and taste claims were offered to 156 German consumers wearing eye-tracking glasses. The researchers found that consumers looked at health claims longer than nutrition or taste claims. Nonetheless, when it came to purchase, consumers more often bought orange juice labelled with the nutrition claim and milk chocolate labelled with the taste claim. Consumers apply their own set of criteria when selecting products to purchase and understanding the principles behind that selection for different consumer segments is important for developing novel functional foods. Depending on the product category, the eye-tracking methodology can be successfully used to craft food claims for functional foods, with consumers' needs and expectations in mind.

Case study based on Steinhauser et al. (2019).

4.5 Combination of different methodological approaches

Those developing new foods should seek to use a range of consumer insight methodologies to understand consumer behaviours and motivations, trade-offs, value propositions to design products that closely meet consumer expectations. Some of the methodologies can be used at the product ideation, or design stages, and others at the stage of understanding what attributes are driving consumer preferences. The type of functional foods being developed, and the information required to make strategic business decisions, dictates the combination of methodologies that can be used by product developers (Fig. 4.1). Combinations of various methodologies, quantitative and qualitative, sensory and statistical, can offer more comprehensive insights to guide the NPD process.

4.6 Conclusions and implications for functional food product development

In this chapter and the previous one, we have noted the significance of a market-oriented approach to the NPD process, which is linked to higher profitability and success at developing new products. Being market-oriented means engaging the consumer and generating insights to drive the NPD process. In fact, as Alongi and Anese (2021) note, the consumer is often used for the prototyping and launch stages, rather than the ideation and concept design stages.

We outlined the various market-oriented research methodologies that food firms can use to develop more successful functional foods, which closely meet consumer needs. This market-oriented approach to NPD in the functional foods' category is more relevant due to the complexity of marketing science to consumers and the range of food choice factors that influence consumers in relation to functional foods. This is also true as science identifies new benefits of existing ingredients, or identifies the benefits of new ingredients, and firms seek to commercialise the science through new functional foods in competitive markets.

In relation to developing new functional foods, product developers might use different combinations of the various methodologies we have outlined in these chapters to understand consumers, in terms of producing new functional foods. These products could be for different consumer segments (e.g., the elderly or gluten-free), new categories of functional foods (e.g., meat-free alternatives, nutrition for individuals, or personalised

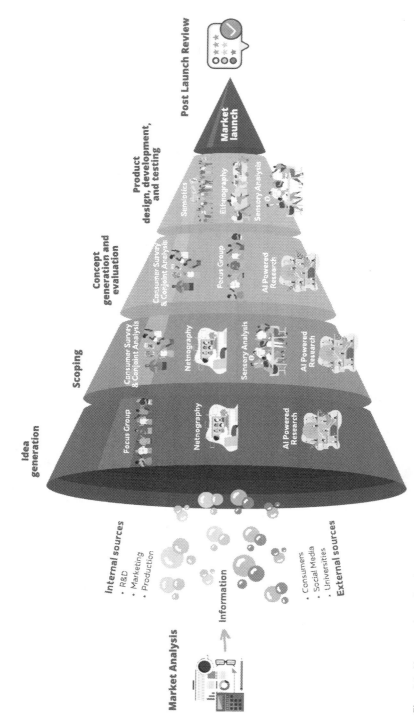

Fig. 4.1 *New product development and market-oriented consumer insights methodologies for functional foods.* *Source:* Authors based on Chesbrough (2020), Cooper (2006), and Relich (2021). Created using Canva Pro. Art elements: artbesouro and Sketchify.

Table 4.3 An interactive overview of different methodologies for gaining consumer insights on functional foods.

Methodology	Data type	Key strengths	Key weaknesses	Knowledge level	Technology cost	Time cost	Self-evaluation for your research: suitable/doable[a]
Focus group discussion	QUAL	Participant discussion	Unpredictable group dynamics and digressions	Medium	Low	Medium	
Ethnography	QUAL	In-depth, detailed insights	Complexity and access to participants	High	Medium	High	
Netnography	QUAL/ QUAN	Insights into online communities	Ethics and data protection issues	Medium	Medium	Medium	
Semiotics	QUAL/ QUAN	Preferences for packaging design; brand management directions	Requires design experience and selection of correct target market	Medium	Medium	Medium	**Scenarios** (Suitable/Doable): • Yes/Yes → **Proceed** • No/No → **Stop** • Yes/No → **Fix or Stop** • No/Yes → **Stop**
Sensory analysis	QUAL/ QUAN	Acceptance of a product's sensory profile and consumer preferences	Prior knowledge, controlled site and recruitment	High	Medium to high	Medium to high	
Consumer survey/ conjoint analysis	QUAN	Consumer preferences, trade-offs and segments	Statistical and econometric skills required	Medium/ High	Low/ Medium	Low/ Medium	
New technologies: Big Data, mobile apps and eye tracking	QUAL/ QUAN	Advanced level of data gained using technology	Cost of technology	High	High	Medium	

Source: Authors.
[a]Note: "Suitable" refers to whether the methodology and its data type suit the research objectives and questions, and the stage of the NPD process. "Doable" refers to whether the researcher/team possesses the needed knowledge level and could invest in the required technology and time. "Fix" means to cover the gap in what is "Doable" by sourcing the required knowledge and/or technology; and/or time (if successful, then it translates into Yes/Yes→Proceed scenario).

nutrition) or with sustainability as a value proposition. Valera and Ares (2018) noted there should be more interdisciplinary and realistic research to tackle complex questions underlying food behaviours and consumer perceptions. In addition, getting the market and technical functions to work closely together in organisations builds on another key identified NPD success factor across food products: a multidisciplinary approach to NPD. The importance of closely meeting consumer expectations, through product design, increases in more competitive markets, where consumers are faced with a wide range of choices, brands, and influences from traditional and digital media. Utilising market-oriented methodologies that integrate the consumer into the functional foods NPD process requires various knowledge, time, and technology investments (Table 4.3), but will lead to more successful new products.

References

Alongi, M., Anese, M., 2021. Re-thinking functional food development through a holistic approach. J. Funct. Foods 81, 104466. https://doi.org/10.1016/j.jff.2021.104466.

Aversa, J., Hernandez, T., Doherty, S., 2021. Incorporating big data within retail organizations: a case study approach. Journal of Retailing and Consumer Services 60, 102447. https://doi.org/10.1016/j.jretconser.2021.102447.

Bi, J., Ennis, D.M., 1999. Statistical Models for the A-Not A Method. J. Sens. Stud. 16, 215–237. https://doi.org/10.1111/j.1745-459X.2001.tb00297.x.

Birkin, M., Clarke, G., Corcoran, J., Stimson, R., 2021. Chapter 1: Introduction to big data applications in geography and planning. Birkin, M., Clarke, G., Corcoran, J., Stimson, R. (Eds.). Big Data Applications in Geography and Planning-An Essential Companion. Edward Elgar, Cheltenham, United Kingdom, pp. 1–7.

Blazquez, D., Domenech, J., 2018. Big Data sources and methods for social and economic analyses. Technological Forecasting & Social Change 130, 99–113. https://doi.org/10.1016/j.techfore.2017.07.027.

Bogue, J., Collins, O., Troy, A-J., 2017. Chapter 2: Market analysis and concept development of functional foods. In: Bagchi, D., Nair, S. (Eds.), Developing New Functional Food and Nutraceutical Products. Academic Press, Amsterdam, the Netherlands, pp. 29–45. https://doi.org/10.1016/B978-0-12-802780-6.00002-X.

Cais-Sokolińska, D., Walkowiak-Tomczak, D., 2021. Consumer-perception, nutritional, and functional studies of a yogurt with restructured elderberry juice. J. Dairy Sci. 104 (2), 1318–1335. https://doi.org/10.3168/jds.2020-18770.

Carabante, K.M., Prinyawiwatkul, W., 2018. Data analyses of a multiple-samples sensory ranking test and its duplicated test: a review. J. Sens. Stud. 33, e12435. https://doi.org/10.1111/joss.12435.

Chesbrough, H., 2020. Open Innovation Results: Going Beyond the Hype and Getting Down to Business. Oxford University Press, Oxford, United Kingdom.

Contreras-Rodriguez, O., Mata, F., Verdejo-Román, Ramírez-Bernabé, R., Moreno, D., Vilar-Lopez, R., Soriano-Mas, C., Verdejo- García, A., 2020. Neural-based valuation of functional foods among lean and obese individuals. Nutr. Res. 78, 27–35. https://doi.org/10.1016/j.nutres.2020.03.006.

Cooper, R.G., 2006. *The seven principles of the latest Stage-Gate® method add up to a streamlined, new product idea-to-launch process.* http://www.five-is.com/wp-content/uploads/2013/12/Cooper_2006_Formula_for_Success.pdf (accessed March 19, 2021).

Crucean, D., Debucquet, G., Rannou, C., le-Bail, A., le-Bail, P., 2019. Vitamin B4 as a salt substitute in bread: a challenging and successful new strategy. Sensory perception and acceptability by French consumers. Appetite 134, 17–25. https://doi.org/10.1016/j.appet.2018.12.020.

De Farias Silva, C.E., Correia Vieira, R., Caetano da Silva, I.C., Barbosa e Oliveria Cerqueira, R., Pereira Andrade, N., Claudino da Silva, F., Pimentel de Andrade, F., de Souza Abud, A.K., Andreola, K., Pereira Taranto, O., 2021. Combining fruit pulp and rice protein agglomerated with collagen to potentialize it as a functional food: particle characterization, pulp formulation and sensory analysis. J. Food Sci. Technol. 58, 4194–4204 doi:10.1007/s13197-020-04892-7.

Dehlholm, C., Brockhoff, P.B., Meinert, L., Aaslying, M.D., Bredie, WL.P., 2012. Rapid descriptive sensory methods-comparison of free multiple sorting, partial napping, napping, flash profiling and conventional profiling. Food Qual. Preference 26, 267–277. http://dx.doi.org/10.1016/j.foodqual.2012.02.012.

Erevelles, S., Fukawa, N., Swayne, L., 2016. Big data consumer analytics and the transformation of marketing. Journal of Business Research 69 (2), 897–904. http://dx.doi.org/10.1016/j.jbusres.2015.07.001.

Geisen, E., Romano Bergstrom, J., 2017. Chapter 5: Developing the usability testing protocol. Usability Testing for Survey Research. Morgan Kaufmann, Cambridge, MA, pp. 111–129. https://doi.org/10.1016/B978-0-12-803656-3.00005-1.

Green, P.E., Rao, V.R., 1971. Conjoint measurement for quantifying judgmental data. Journal of Marketing Research 8 (3), 355–363. https://doi.org/10.2307/3149575.

Hamilton, L.M., Lahne, J., 2020. Fast and automated sensory analysis: using natural language processing for descriptive lexicon development. Food Qual. Preference 83, 103926. https://doi.org/10.1016/j.foodqual.2020.103926.

Hofacker, C.F., Malthouse, E.C., Sultan, F., 2016. Big data and consumer behaviour: imminent opportunities. Journal of Consumer Marketing 33 (2), 89–97. https://doi.org/10.1108/JCM-04-2015-1399.

Huang, J., Peng, Y., Wan, X., 2021. The color-flavor incongruency effect in visual search for food labels: an eye-tracking study. Food Qual. Preference 88, 104078. https://doi.org/10.1016/j.foodqual.2020.104078.

Huang, L., Bai, L., Gong, S., 2020. The effects of carrier, benefit, and perceived trust in information channel on functional food purchase intention among Chinese consumers. Food Qual. Preference 81, 103854. https://doi.org/10.1016/j.foodqual.2019.103854.

Kemp, S.E., Ng, M., Hollowood, T., Hort, J., 2018. Chapter 1: Introduction to descriptive analysis. In: Kemp, S.E., Hort, J., Hollowood, T. (Eds.), Descriptive Analysis in Sensory Evaluation. Wiley-Blackwell, Hoboken, NJ, pp. 3–39.

Lawless, H.T., Heymann, H., 2010. Chapter 1: Introduction. Sensory Evaluation of Food - Principles and Practices, Food Science Text Series. Springer, New York, NY, pp. 1–18.

Lazer, D., Kennedy, R., King, G., Vespignani, A., 2014. The parable of Google Flu: traps in big data analysis. Science 343 (6176), 1203–1205. https://doi.org/10.1126/science.1248506.

Lutz, C.R., 2021. Exploring Conjoint Analysis. Qualtrics, Provo, UT.

Matz, S., Netzer, O., 2017. Using Big Data as a window into consumers' psychology. Current Opinions in Behavioral Sciences 18, 7–12. http://dx.doi.org/10.1016/j.cobeha.2017.05.009.

McCrickerd, K., Forde, C., 2016. Sensory influences on food intake control: moving beyond palatability. Obes. Rev. 17, 18–29. https://doi.org/10.1111/obr.12340.

Mellentin, J., 2009. Failures in Functional Foods and Beverages-and What They Reveal About Success. New Nutrition Business, London, United Kingdom.

Michail, N., 2016. FoodProfiler: The NPD app that tracks the 'what, when and why' of consumer food choices. https://www.foodnavigator.com/article/2016/08/29/food-profiler-the-npd-app-that-tracks-the-what-when-and-why-of-consumer-food-choices (accessed June 17, 2021).

Michell, K.A., Isweiri, H., Newman, S.E., Bunning, M., Bellows, L.L., Dinges, M., Grabos, L.E., Rao, S., Foster, M.T., Heuberger, A.L., Prenni, J.E., Thompson, H.J., Uchanski, M.E., Weir, T.L., Johnson, S.A., 2020. Microgreens: consumer sensory perception and acceptance of an emerging functional food crop. J. Food Sci. 85 (4), 926–935. https://doi.org/10.1111/1750-3841.15075.

Nan, X., Verrill, L., Iles, I., 2017. As much calcium as a glass of milk! Understanding American consumers' preferences for fortified foods. Journal of Food Products Marketing 23 (1), 24–41. https://doi.org/10.1080/10454446.2017.1244782.

Nystrand, B.T., Olsen, S.O., 2020. Consumers' attitudes and intentions toward consuming functional foods in Norway. Food Qual. Preference 80, 103827. https://doi.org/10.1016/j.foodqual.2019.103827.

Orme, B.K., 2010. Getting Started with Conjoint Analysis: Strategies for Product Design and Pricing Research. Research Publishers LLC, Madison, WI.

O'Sullivan, M.G., 2017. Chapter 1: Difference methods. In: O'Sullivan, M.G. (Ed.), A Handbook for Sensory and Consumer-Driven New Product Development - Innovative Technologies for the Food and Beverage Industry. Woodhead Publishing Series in Food Science, Technology and Nutrition. Elsevier, Cambridge, United Kingdom. pp. 3–12. https://doi.org/10.1016/C2014-0-03843-9.

Pantano, E., Dennis, C., De, P.M., 2021. Shopping centres revisited: the interplay between consumers' spontaneous online communications and retail planning. Journal of Retailing and Consumer Services 61, 102576. https://doi.org/10.1016/j.jretconser.2021.102576.

Park, E., 2019. The role of satisfaction on consumer reuse to airline services: an application of Big Data approaches. Journal of Retailing and Consumer Studies 47, 370–374. https://doi.org/10.1016/j.jretconser.2019.01.004.

Petit, O., Javornik, A., Velasco, C., 2021. We eat first with our (digital) eyes: enhancing mental simulation of eating experiences via visual-enabling technologies. Journal of Retailing. https://doi.org/10.1016/j.jretai.2021.04.003.

Peng-Li, D., Mathiesen, S.L., Chan, R.C.K., Byrne, D.V., Wang, Q.J., 2021. Sounds healthy: modelling sound-evoked consumer food choice through visual attention. Appetite 164, 105264. https://doi.org/10.1016/j.appet.2021.105264.

Peryam, D.R., Pilgrim, F.J., Peterson, M.S., 1954. Food acceptance testing methodology. Journal of Association of Official Agricultural Chemists 38 (4), 1022. https://doi.org/10.1093/jaoac/38.4.1022.

Piggott, J.R., Simpson, S.J., Williams, S.A.R., 1998. Sensory Analysis. Int. J. Food Sci. Technol. 33, 7–18. https://doi.org/10.1046/j.1365-2621.1998.00154.x.

Porretta, S., 2021. Chapter 1: Food development: the sensory and consumer approach. In: Porretta, S., Moskowitz, H., Gere, A. (Eds.), Consumer-based New Product Development for the Food Industry. The Royal Society of Chemistry, Croydon, United Kingdom, pp. 3–20.

Punter, P.H., 2018. Chapter 13: Free choice profiling. In: Kemp, S.E., Hort, J., Hollowood, T. (Eds.). Descriptive Analysis in Sensory Evaluation. Wiley-Blackwell, Hoboken, NJ/Chichester, United Kingdom, pp. 513–533. https://doi.org/10.1002/9781118991657.ch13.

Puurtinen, M., Hoppu, U., Puputti, S., Mattila, S., Sandell, M., 2021. Investigation visual attention toward foods in a salad buffet with mobile eye tracking. Food Qual. Preference 93, 104290. https://doi.org/10.1016/j.foodqual.2021.104290.

Rao, V.R., 2014. Applied Conjoint Analysis. Springer-Verlag, Berlin and Heidelberg, Germany. https://doi.org/10.1007/978-3-540-87753-0.

Rebouças, M.C., do Carmo Passos Rodrigues, M., Burnier Arcanjo Ferreira, B., De Freitas, S.M., 2020. Evaluation of the effect of label attributes over the purchase intention of a cashew nut functional beverage using conjoint analysis. Food Sci. Technol. Int. 27 (2), 164–171. https://doi.org/10.1177/1082013220942434.

Relich, M., 2021. Chapter 1: Product development: state of the art and challenges. Decision Support for Product Development: Using Computational Intelligence for information Acquisition in Enterprise Databases. Springer Nature, Cham, Switzerland, pp. 1–26. https://doi.org/10.1007/978-3-030-43897-5_1#DOI.

Samala, N., Sama, V., 2018. A study on food ordering mobile apps. Asian Journal of Research in Social Sciences and Humanities 8 (7), 10–23. http://dx.doi.org/10.5958/2249-7315.2018.00108.9.

Samoggia, A., Riedel, B., 2020. Assessment of nutrition-focused mobile apps' influence on consumers' healthy food behaviour and nutrition knowledge. Food Res. Int. 128, 1087766. https://doi.org/10.1016/j.foodres.2019.108766.

Srinivasan, V., Park, C.S., 1997. Surprising robustness of the self-explicated approach to consumer preference structure measurement. Journal of Marketing Research 34 (2), 286–291. https://doi.org/10.2307/3151865.

Steinhauser, J., Janssen, M., Hamm, U., 2019. Consumers' purchase decisions for products with nutrition and health claims: What role do product category and gaze duration on claims play? Appetite 141, 104337. https://doi.org/10.1016/j.appet.2019.104337.

Stone, H., Sidel, J.L., 2004. Sensory Evaluation Practices. Elsevier Academic Press, San Diego, CA/London, United Kingdom.

Tian, G., Lu, L., McIntosh, C., 2021. What factors affects customers' dining sentiments and their ratings: evidence from restaurant online review data. Food Qual. Preference 88, 104060. https://doi.org/10.1016/j.foodqual.2020.104060.

Torri, L., Tuccillo, F., Bonelli, S., Piraino, S., Leone, A., 2020. The attitudes of Italian consumers towards jellyfish as novel food. Food Qual. Preference 79, 103782. https://doi.org/10.1016/j.foodqual.2019.103782.

Valera, P., Ares, G., 2018. Chapter 1: Recent advances in consumer science. In: Ares, G., Varela, P. (Eds.), *Methods in Consumer Research*, Volume 1, New Approaches to Classic Methods. Woodhead Publishing Series in Food Science, Technology and Nutrition. Elsevier, Cambridge, United Kingdom, pp. 49–77. https://doi.org/10.1016/B978-0-08-102089-0.00001-7.

Velázquez, A.L., Alcaire, F., Vidal, L., Varela, P., Næs, T., Ares, G., 2021. The influence of label information on the snacks parents choose for their children: Individual differences in a choice based conjoint test. Food Qual. Preference 94, 104296. https://doi.org/10.1016/j.foodqual.2021.104296.

CHAPTER 5

Competitive advantage through multidisciplinary innovation in nutraceuticals: From concept optimisation to context transformation

Stefan Korber[a], Frank Siedlok[b], Lisa Callagher[a], Ziad Elsahn[c]
[a]University of Auckland, New Zealand
[b]Heriot-Watt University, Edinburgh, United Kingdom
[c]Northumbria University, Newcastle Business School, United Kingdom

5.1 Introduction

Multidisciplinary collaboration[a] in academic research and organisational settings is increasingly seen as imperative for developing innovative solutions that meet current and future customer needs and for solving the complex problems that contemporary societies face (Dell'Era, 2009; Ibert and Mueller, 2015; Rhoten, 2004; Siedlok and Hibbert, 2014). The integration of a broad base of knowledge and practices is particularly important for developing and commercializing consumer-oriented nutraceuticals and functional foods (NFFs) (Bröring, 2013; Galati et al., 2016). Companies that operate in these sectors span traditional knowledge boundaries (e.g., pharmacology, chemistry, and nutritional science) and must align their products with customers' ever-changing concerns and expectations (Bröring et al., 2006; Bröring and Cloutier, 2008). Further, NFFs have been lauded for their potential to alleviate pressing problems such as malnutrition and obesity (Siedlok et al., 2010; Sijtsema et al., 2020). To maximise the value that NFFs generate, Alongi and Anese (2021) argued that NFFs should adopt

---

[a]The terms cross-disciplinary, multidisciplinary, multidisciplinary, and transdisciplinary are often used interchangeably in NFF literature. We use the term "multidisciplinary" because it typically refers to all collaborations and interactions among epistemological boundaries. For a discussion of the distinctions among these concepts, see Huutoniemi et al. (2010) and Siedlok and Hibbert (2014).

Case Studies on the Business of Nutraceuticals, Functional and Super Foods
DOI: https://doi.org/10.1016/B978-0-12-821408-4.00007-9

multidisciplinary approaches and involve a broader range of stakeholders including "food technologists, nutritionists, clinicians, marketing experts, as well as consumers, with different interests, perspectives, and skills that can hardly be matched" (p. 8).

While multidisciplinarity is often mentioned as vital for NFFs, accounts of what disciplines are brought together and for what purpose remain anecdotal (see, Sijtsema et al., 2020 for an exception). In particular, extant research has not adequately addressed two interrelated questions. First, while scholars acknowledge that multidisciplinary approaches can enhance the competitiveness of NFF firms by enabling them to innovate, it does not specify how these firms can differentiate themselves from competitors through multidisciplinarity (Galati et al., 2016; Sijtsema et al., 2020). Second, existing accounts remain focused on "narrow" forms of multidisciplinarity that are predominantly confined to knowledge and practices related to Science, Technology, Engineering, and Medicine/Mathematics (STEM).

Although STEM disciplines are valuable to NFF firms, science- and technology-centred solutions often fail to meet customer needs and seldom tackle complex social problems (Fischer et al., 2011). In turn, calls for wider multidisciplinary approaches that involve knowledge and methods from "conceptually diverse fields that cross the boundaries of broad intellectual areas" (Huutoniemi et al., 2010, p. 82) require knowledge and practices beyond STEM. In particular, knowledge, skills, and methods that originate in HASS (humanities, arts, and social sciences) are increasingly seen as relevant to STEM-based research and to technology and science-driven organisations (Fischer et al., 2011; Hartley, 2016). Yet, whether and how the scope of multidisciplinarity (narrow vs wide) affects the competitive advantage of NFF firms remains unclear. In turn, we ask:

How do narrow and wide forms of multidisciplinary collaborations contribute to strategic innovation in nutraceutical organisations?

To address this question, we integrate two literature. First, we use strategic innovation literature to theorise how organisations can create sustainable competitive advantage through new products, services, and business models (Markides, 1997; Talke et al., 2011). They can do so through search (Gavetti et al., 2017) for sustainable opportunities via internal R&D, open collaboration (e.g., with research institutes), or superior capabilities that make it possible to continuously scan and exploit exogenous market dynamics (e.g., changing customer preferences). Strategic innovation in NFF firms can also refer to proactively shaping (Gavetti et al., 2017) the business context in which a firm operates (e.g., through lobbying for regulatory changes or influencing expectations and behaviours of customers or other stakeholders). Second, we use research on multidisciplinarity (Carlile, 2002; Klein, 2017), which shows that the benefits (and challenges) of multidisciplinary collaboration depend on the "scope" of multidisciplinarity (Huutoniemi et al., 2010). This lens lets us distinguish between "narrow" and "wide" multidisciplinarity, depending on the combability and complementarity of worldviews, knowledge, and methods used. To date, the evidence that narrow and broad forms contribute to distinct shaping- and search-oriented strategic innovation by NFF firms remains anecdotal.

We first outline the lenses underlying our research and introduce a theoretical framework that guides our subsequent analysis. After that, we present our findings and discuss case studies that illustrate four different modes of multidisciplinary innovation in NFF firms, their relevance for a firm's competitive advantage, the challenges and shortfalls associated with each mode, and their potential impact on society. We conclude with implications for decision-makers regarding the need to integrate a broader set of knowledge and practices in their innovation processes and caution against instrumental forms of multidisciplinarity.

5.2 The importance of multidisciplinarity for strategic innovation

In this section, we outline extant perspectives on strategic innovation and multidisciplinary collaboration and their importance for NFF firms. We then develop a theoretical framework that integrates these perspectives and guides our analysis.

5.2.1 Strategic innovation orientation: Product optimisation versus context transformation

Knowledge and innovation are critical to firms' efforts to achieve growth, profitability, and competitive advantage (Gavetti, 2017). A firm's innovation orientation guides its strategy and "reflects the firm's philosophy of how to manage innovation through a deeply rooted set of values and beliefs that guide firm-wide innovation activity" (Talke et al., 2011, p. 821).

In a recent review, Gavetti et al. (2017) argue that many scholars have examined how firms use search to pursue strategic innovation by identifying and exploiting profit opportunities "in exogenously-determined business contexts" (Gavetti et al., 2017, p. 195). Search can focus on developing innovations through R&D and identifying and exploiting present or emerging customer needs (Kodama and Shibata, 2014; Talke et al., 2011). Its success depends on an organisation's capabilities to orchestrate internal and external R&D, to constantly monitor exogenous changes in competition, customers, and technology and to capitalize on emerging opportunities (Markides, 1997; Tripsas and Gavetti, 2000). This literature suggests several ways multidisciplinary approaches can catalyse search-focused strategic innovation.

First, multidisciplinarity may enhance an innovation's novelty and help firms optimise technical aspects related to new products and services. For example, multidisciplinary collaboration can help NFF firms overcome "theoretical and technological problems" (Galati et al., 2016, p. 17) in product development, to optimise intrinsic product characteristics (e.g., storability and health benefits), and to facilitate improvements in operational processes (Bigliardi and Galati, 2013; Galati et al., 2016). Second, multidisciplinarity is associated with closer customer orientation and an empathetic understanding of market needs (Matthyssens et al., 2008; Sijtsema et al., 2020). For example, Talke et al. (2011) found top management teams that have more diverse educational, functional, industry, and organisational backgrounds are more likely to have a market-focused (instead of a technology-focused) orientation to strategic innovation, which they define as a "firm's posture towards creating an understanding of its customers and serving customer needs" (Talke et al., 2011, p. 821). Bogue et al. (2017) thus urged NFF firms to adopt multidisciplinary approaches in new product development because "they can assist firms to manage knowledge more effectively and efficiently and develop more market-oriented food products that gain consumer acceptance" (p. 42).

While a search perspective takes an external business context (e.g., customer preferences or regulatory frameworks) as given, Gavetti et al. (2017) note an alternative path in which firms "attempt to shape the context in which they do business in pursuits of competitive advantage"(p. 195). Shaping activities can involve lobbying for favourable policy, knowledge dissemination related to new technologies, or efforts to transform customer perceptions and expectations (Gavetti et al., 2017). Given the importance of customer perceptions and regulatory frameworks for NFFs, shaping strategies are particularly relevant for NFF firms (Matthyssens et al., 2008). For instance, Almeida et al. (2014) examine how Danone shaped new values and collective concerns regarding food functionality and created favourable regulations by engaging with government agencies and politicians. While the literature pays scant attention to how multidisciplinary approaches contributed to search-oriented strategic innovation, it offers some hints. For example, non-technical experts can help firms shape customer perspectives through tailored messaging (Almeida et al., 2014), help shape regulatory frameworks (Khan et al., 2013; Ritvala and Granqvist, 2009), and help transform stakeholders' behaviours and concerns (Frewer et al., 2003).

Further, the literature has paid little attention to the scope of multidisciplinarity that collaborative engagements entail (Huutoniemi et al., 2010, p. 82).

5.2.2 Scope of multidisciplinarity: narrow versus wide

The success of multidisciplinary collaborations depends on the compatibility of worldviews, knowledge, and methods of inquiry used by the involved actors (Carlile, 2002; Klein, 2017; Siedlok and Hibbert, 2014). Natural sciences are typically associated with a positivist worldview wherein a single (objective) reality is thought to explain empirical phenomena. Such assumptions are reflected in STEM methods aimed at discovering causal explanations through deductive reasoning and experiments (McGregor, 2015). In contrast, HASS often uses an interpretivist paradigm wherein (social) reality can be understood only from the perspective of social actors and the varied socio-cultural forces that shape—and are shaped by—social beings (Wierzbicka, 2011). These assumptions give rise to more inductive modes of inquiry that emphasise peculiar and singular events—historic battles, works of art, texts, and observations—that are integrated and interpreted to understand larger socio-cultural "wholes" (Holm et al., 2015). Depending on the relative compatibility in worldviews, knowledge, and methods, the literature distinguishes between "narrow" and "broad" multidisciplinarity (Huutoniemi et al., 2010; Klein, 2017).

"Narrow" multidisciplinarity refers to collaborations where "participating fields are conceptually close to each other, typically representing the same broad domain of scholarly work" (Huutoniemi et al., 2010, p. 82). In such instances, the methods and worldviews of involved actors are relatively compatible. Examples include collaborations that rely on knowledge and practices grounded in STEM disciplines (Huutoniemi et al., 2010). Such narrow forms of multidisciplinarity, like those involving pharmaceutical experts, nutritional scientists, and process engineers, dominate the literature on NFF (e.g., Boehlje and Bröring, 2011; Ciliberti et al., 2016). Nonetheless, technology and science-focused innovation can fail both to meet customer expectations and to maximise the social, economic, and environmental impact of solutions (Khan et al., 2013; Sankaran and Mouly, 2007).

To address these shortcomings, the literature highlights the benefits of broad multidisciplinary collaborations that integrate "conceptually diverse fields" spanning broad intellectual areas (Fischer et al., 2011; Klein, 2017). Recently, practitioners and academics have attempted to bridge the gap between HASS and STEM disciplines (Hartley, 2016). While references to "broad" multidisciplinary endeavours in NFF firms are scant, anecdotal evidence hints at several potential benefits. First, during new product development, broad multidisciplinarity approaches can enhance creativity and enable cultural and technical knowledge to be recombined in the ideation process (Sankaran and Mouly, 2007). For instance, Liufu (2020, p. 351) argued that the conception of an idea for a new functional food may begin in archaeology, history, and anthropology, which traditionally lies outside of the traditional realm of science. Looking into other cultures or into the past can provide invaluable information about foods or compounds that have been deemed to result in a positive health benefit.

Second, HASS-based practices can generate insights into latent needs and social or cultural trends, fostering customer-oriented product development (Matthyssens et al., 2008; Szerszynski and Galarraga, 2013). Alongi and Anese (2021) argued that marketing surveys to collect quantitative information on consumer attitudes about NFF "should be merged with social and cultural aspects by an anthropological approach" (p. 9). Third, broad multidisciplinarity involving a range of stakeholders can enhance innovations' impact and facilitate positive transformation through multiactor and multidisciplinary collaboration (Ritvala and Granqvist, 2009). For instance, Siedlok et al. (2010) claimed that "scientifically proved benefits of such products [NFF], combined with policy support and mass education and policy from governments, might help to combat the health concerns of modern societies" (p. 579).

5.2.3 An integrative framework

The literature on innovation and NFF emphasise that multidisciplinarity approaches can catalyse strategic innovation, but they suggest that the results of these endeavours will depend on the disciplinary distance of the actors involved. Fig. 5.1 integrates the literature on strategic innovation and the potential scopes of multidisciplinarity to offer a more cohesive account.

Search-focused strategic innovation (Gavetti et al., 2017; Markides, 1997) entails activities that enable NFF firms to gain competitive advantage

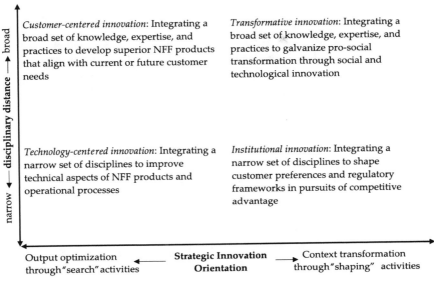

Fig. 5.1 *Integrative framework.*

through "a superior product strategy, juggling ingredients, technology, and labelling to optimise the product portfolio" (International, 2015). In this context, narrow forms of multidisciplinarity are usually related to technology-centred innovation that attempts to optimise the intrinsic aspects of products or operational processes. In contrast, "broad" multidisciplinarity spans social and natural sciences have been shown to facilitate customer-centred innovation in NFF and enhance the competitive advantage of NFF firms by facilitating "institutional innovation" that attempts to shape regulatory frameworks and market preferences (Hargrave and Van De Ven, 2006; Kalaitzandonakes, 2000). While institutional innovation is usually associated with economic benefits, broad multidisciplinary collaborations can enable transformative social innovation that maximises social, economic, and benefits by mobilising collective action towards pro-social transformation (Ritvala and Granqvist, 2009).

The four modes in Fig. 5.1 can overlap. Search activities can complement shaping activities. Similarly, like Huutoniemi et al. (2010), we acknowledge "that conceptual distance is not a straightforward property and definitely not a binary variable" and "that even the coarse distinction between narrow and broad scope is informative" (p. 82). While collaborations that bridge HASS and STEM disciplines might imply a "broad" scope, closer attention to the worldviews and methods of the disciplines involved is necessary. For example, while NFF firms often use approaches rooted in business and economics, such endeavours are arguably narrow because they rely on deductive reasoning and quantification. Indeed, lligan (1987, p. 593) labels business studies as "almost entirely science-based education". Others lament that such approaches fail to consider knowledge and methods developed in the arts and humanities (Olmos-Penuela et al., 2014). Reflecting this concern, our conception of "broad" multidisciplinarity in Fig. 5.1 moves beyond business-related knowledge and practices. Instead, we focus on the value of inductive and interpretivist approaches from disciplines like anthropology, philosophy, history, and literature.

5.3 Findings

In this section, we discuss four modes of multidisciplinarity innovation identified in Fig. 5.1, their relevance for a firm's competitive advantage, the challenges involved, and their potential impact on society. To support our arguments, and to emphasise the relevance to NFF firms, we integrate case studies with extant research. We chose these cases for illustrative purposes. They represent the increasing range of NFF firms.

5.3.1 Science and technology-focused innovation

Most literature on multidisciplinary approaches regarding NFF refers to "narrow" forms of integration that are grounded in STEM-based knowledge and practices. NFF development and commercialisation requires expertise in food- and medical-sciences, process engineering, and technology (Mark-Herbert, 2004). These disciplines help firms develop superior product characteristics and to optimise manufacturing and logical processes (Alongi and Anese, 2021; Santini et al., 2018). A multidisciplinary approach can also be useful if legislative frameworks require evidence to support health claims (Alongi and Anese, 2021; Santini et al., 2018). Further, the integration of expertise related to AI and Big Data analytics is framed as increasingly relevant for ingredient discovery, product development, and market research (Sreejith, 2021).

Consider, for instance, Arepa, an NNF based in New Zealand that develops nutraceuticals to aid mental clarity. Its main product uses pine extract, blackcurrant extract, and green tea extract to enhance cognitive functioning. Arepa built a multidisciplinary team to create scientifically proven products and to increase their commercial viability by integrating consumer and medical research. By combining scientists from neuroscience, engineering, food technology, and psychopharmacology with the cofounders' finance and industrial design expertise, Arepa can identify changing customer expectations and formulate a value proposition that addresses those needs. Further, this approach allowed Arepa to scientifically validate its value proposition and to differentiate its product from competing energy drinks.[b]

Such narrow forms of multidisciplinary collaboration may be straightforward because the worldviews of STEM disciplines are broadly aligned (Huutoniemi et al., 2010; Klein, 2017). As such, multidisciplinarity depends on mechanisms to identify relevant partners, establish and manage collaborations, and clarify intellectual property issues (Galati et al., 2016). However, technology-centred innovation (elsewhere termed as technology-push, for example, van Kleef et al., 2002) may fail because it does not consider or understand socio-cultural elements (Chiesa and Frattini, 2011). For example, Bogue et al. (2017) suggested that high failure rates (70%–90%) in NFF development "suggest that many new functional foods have not met with acceptance or consumers have not fully understood the product concept on offer to them" (p. 32). Thus, NFF firms such as Arepa that seek strategic differentiation by investing in R&D and scientific validation may create products that are misaligned with what the market values.

5.3.2 Customer-centred innovation

To address the shortfalls of technology-push innovation, methods and knowledge that originate in the arts and humanities (e.g., ethnography) may help NFF development and commercialisation (Sankaran and Mouly, 2007). HASS-based approaches are presumed to function as "a 'mouthpiece' for society, providing insight into human values and behaviour" (Lowe et al., 2013, p. 208) and to enable customer-centred innovation. Yet, there are various mechanisms and tools for achieving this goal. The literature on innovation in NFF firms usually refers to the adoption of frameworks like design thinking (Sijtsema et al., 2020; Tkaczewska et al., 2021) that use methods from the Humanities (e.g., anthropology) and the arts (e.g., visual design) and involve deep engagement with

[b]On its website (https://drinkarepa.com), Arepa notes that its products are based upon "neuroscience not pseudoscience" and provides references to academic publications that support these claims.

customers during product ideation and development. More substantial forms of broad multidisciplinarity can involve specialists or prolonged collaborations that span disciplinary boundaries. For example, research in ethno-pharmacology and ethno-botany integrates social and historical knowledge with food and medical science and can inform ingredient discovery and concept development in NFF innovation (Huntington, 2000; Sankaran and Mouly, 2007).

There are, however, few substantial examples of such broad integration; it is unclear how and whether NFF firms engage deeply with socio and cultural aspects. Similarly, Sankaran and Mouly (2007) noted that "the ethnographic component of most published ethno-pharmacology has been deemed to be weak, if not non-existent" (p. 340). Potential exceptions are collaborative engagements in New Zealand that integrate indigenous (Māori) knowledge, "western" science, and business expertise. For instance, a project titled "Mamaku Whakaoraora" (the indigenous name for a tree fern) seeks to explore and exploit the commercial potential of tree ferns that the Maori have used as food and medicine. According to the project description, the research constitutes a transcultural inquiry and melds Māori knowledge and capabilities with western science and technology.[c] This project involves close engagement with Māori scientists and businesses to turn cultural knowledge into commercial opportunities.

Apart from such exceptions, attempts to integrate HASS-based knowledge in NPD seem limited to superficial borrowing of concepts and tools such as Design Thinking (Siedlok and Hibbert, 2014). Yet, the unreflective adoption of such tools may fail to provide "deep insights" or to improve innovation quality (Iskander, 2018; Seidel and Fixson, 2013). Indeed, Rao (2018) dismisses design thinking companies like IDEO as "drive-by" anthropology, where designers never fully immerse themselves in their subjects' world. More substantive forms of integration, such as that of Mamaku Whakaoraora, come with their own challenges. For example, inductive and cultural methods of knowledge generation are often at odds with deductive reasoning and quantification and are often subordinate to scientific and technological approaches. They hence have little impact on dominant practices or knowledge and often fail to translate social aspects into meaningful change (Klein, 2017). In particular, innovation approaches that focus on meeting current customer needs might fail to

[c]https://waateanews.com/2019/11/01/mamaku-project-offers-hope-for-puku-diseases/.

deliver positive outcomes for a broader range of stakeholders and to gal-vanise behavioural changes.

5.3.3 Institutional innovation

Under labels such as "institutional innovation" (Hargrave and Van De Ven, 2006) or "institutional entrepreneurship" (Almeida et al., 2014), recent literature emphasises how NFF firms can gain competitive advantage by attempting to shape the socio-economic context in which they operate. They can do so through isolated efforts or, more commonly, through collective action at the industry level (Mark-Herbert, 2004).

For example, Oatly, the world's largest and original oat milk company, was founded by brothers Rickard (a food scientist) and Bjorn (a software engineer) Öste in 1993 to provide a healthier, more sustainable alternative to cow's milk for lactose-intolerant individuals. Oatly uses an enzymatic production process that turns oats into nutritious, dairy-free, food, and beverages (Oatly Group AB, 2020). As of December 31, 2020, Oatly's products were available in approximately 60,000 retail outlets and 32,200 coffee shops in more than 20 countries. According to the founders, Oatly (and a second venture, Aventure) are based on the "commercial potential [of] forming multidisciplinary groups to develop innovative food products with unique properties" (Aventure, 2021). By assembling a team of food-processing engineers, medical and enzyme experts, and environmental scientists Oatly can develop superior products and scientifically validate its health and environmental claims (Koch, 2020).

Some evidence suggests that Oatly's competitive advantage extends beyond its product characteristics. Oatly is portrayed as a brand that "promote[s] oppositional moralities by actively transforming shared ideals, concerns, or criticisms" and seeks to drive "systemic changes in production and consumption practices" (Koch, 2020, p. 593). Reflecting this image, Oatly's value proposition has shifted from a narrow focus on lactose intoler-ance to a focus on health benefits for a broader set of customers and to the lower environmental impact of oat milk relative to dairy farming. By inte-grating scientific expertise and the sophisticated use of sales and market-ing techniques, Oatly seeks to leverage its value propositions to transform customers' attitudes and concerns (Bocken et al., 2020). Oatly not only markets the scientifically validated health and environmental aspects of a dairy-free diet but also has its representatives give presentations at schools about climate change and food impact and organise training courses for chefs and baristas (Bocken et al., 2020; Koch, 2020). Fuentes and Fuentes (2017) note that Oatly portrays the products and practices of competing industries (dairy milk) as "unethical (animal welfare issues), unsustainable, unhealthy, corporate and non-local" (pp. 544-545). Finally, when Oatly recognised a "problematic regulatory system hindering the growth of the plant-based [products]" (Koch, 2020, p. 600), it began a trade organisation (Plant-based Sweden") to influence policy discussions.

However, such shaping strategies can pose challenges. First, they require substantial investments, relevant networks, and sophisticated skills. Second, other organisations can exploit the changes in consumer behaviour that such strategies evoke. Recently, analysts have questioned Oatly's viability, noting its products lack differentiation from the plethora of new oat milk products in the market (Evans and Terazono, 2021). Further, it is unclear whether a marketing-driven approach can lead to the "systemic changes in production and consumption" (Koch, 2020, p. 593) that Oatly claims to pursue. First, Oatly follows a premium strategy, making its products unaffordable for many. Second, replacing locally produced products (dairy milk) with substitutes that rely on a sophisticated production process and an international supply chain is problematic. Third, there is little evidence that Oatly engages with a broader range of knowledge and expertise to achieve the "systemic shift" that is central to its branding strategy. In contrast, Bocken et al. (2020, p. 1) note that accelerating the transitions towards a sustainable food system will require "strategies to engage different stakeholders, such as government, society, and academia" (p. 1). Similarly, Koch (2020) adds that "a sustainable food future cannot be achieved by relying exclusively on initiating changes in individual consumer behaviour" (p. 604).

5.3.4 Transformative pro-social innovation

Some literature highlights the value of broad multidisciplinary collaboration for shaping-oriented strategic innovation in NFF. For example, Alongi and Anese (2021) argue that "anthropological methodologies should be applied to define the most effective strategies to drive consumer choices" (p. 11). Apart from instrumental multidisciplinarity, the integration of a broader set of knowledge and relevant stakeholders can mobilise collective action and maximise the social, economic, and environmental benefits of science and technology. First, research methods from anthropology can be used to identify social and cultural aspects of food consumption that enable nutrition-based interventions to be tailored to local values and expectations (Tumilowicz et al., 2016). Second, HASS-based approaches can be used to translate scientific discoveries to the wider public (Frewer et al., 2003; Ritvala and Granqvist, 2009). Third, broad multidiplomacy complements technology interventions with educational initiatives and policy changes to integrate NFF innovation and behavioural changes (Siedlok et al., 2010). Reflecting these aspects, Ritvala and Granqvist (2009) show how a community intervention program for preventing heart disease required a multidisciplinary approach where "in addition to medicine, knowledge of sociology, social psychology, and social policy were crucial in creating behaviour modification" (p. 136).

The social enterprise HarvestPlus illustrates the multifaceted aspect of what we term "transformative pro-social innovation". HarvestPlus seeks to address hunger and malnutrition through biofortified nutraceutical crops (e.g., Vitamin A Sweet Potato, Iron Beans, Zinc Wheat). Leveraging multidisciplinary collaborations among agricultural experts, nutritionists, public health specialists, and consumer marketing experts, HarvestPlus develops nutritiously enhanced varieties of staple food crops that can be grown locally. These crops have higher amounts of vitamin A, iron, and zinc to address malnutrition. These collaborations consider nutritional needs (e.g., increased density of micronutrients), consumer requirements (e.g., taste, colour, cooking time), and agricultural needs (e.g., higher yield and climate) during product development (Pineda, 2017). To achieve socio-economic insight, HarvestPlus draws on cultural, historic, and business knowledge by conducting ethnographies and behavioural research. It also works with diverse partners from government, business, and civil society to develop, test, and release biofortified crops; educate farmers and consumers on the benefits of these crops, and build markets to ensure these foods reach as many people as possible (Foley et al., 2021).

While HarvestPlus is a social enterprise, recent evidence suggests that for-profit organisations can galvanise collective action towards behaviours and practices that balance economic, social, and environmental concerns. For example, literature on producer cooperatives suggests how organisations can coordinate multidisciplinary food innovation across knowledge boundaries while facilitating the transition to sustainable production and consumption practices by enrolling and engaging a broader set of stakeholders (author citations).

	Technology-oriented innovation	Costumer-oriented innovation	Instrumental institutional innovation	Transformative humanistic innovation
Disciplinary distance	Narrow (STEM-only)	Broad (HASS and STEM)	Narrow (STEM-only)	Broad (HASS and STEM)
Strategic innovation orientation	Concept optimization: Innovation activities focused on optimizing products or processes		Context transformation: Pro-active efforts to shape business context	
Most common approaches	• Collaboration between food and medical science in product development • Collaboration between science and technology in ingredient discovery and market analytics • Collaboration between science and engineering to optimise manufacturing	• Adoption of human-centred innovation methods and tools (e.g., design thinking) • Focused recruitment or prolonged multidisciplinary collaboration (e.g., ethno-pharmacology)	• Lobbying for regulatory change and mobilizing collective action • Shaping public discourse and educating customers to change collective values and expectations • Problematizing substitute products and organizational practices of competitors	• Communication and translation of science • Ethnographic inquiries to understand socio-cultural peculiarities in consumption and production • Mobilizing and orchestrating collective action through the involvement of a broad set of stakeholders
Benefits or rationale for collaboration	• Improved intrinsic product characteristics and process optimization	• Visual appealing packing and extrinsic (sensory) product characteristics; better understanding of current and emerging customer demands	• Differentiation from substitutes • Increasing demands through changed consumer expectations and attitudes • Favourable legislation and policy	• Complementary, non-instrumental commitment from stakeholders • Maximization of social, economic, and environmental benefits from NFF innovation
Potential shortfalls	• Products might fail to meet market needs; regulatory aspects might not be considered	• Superficial adoption of tools might fail to generate relevant insights • Competitiveness rests on current consumer needs and values	• Changed customer expectations can be exploited by competitors • Change direction rests on the worldview of initiating actor • Potentially limited impact	• Might fail to maximize economic benefits for initiating actor

	Technology-oriented innovation	Costumer-oriented innovation	Instrumental institutional innovation	Transformative humanistic innovation
Main challenges of collaboration	• Collaboration rests mainly on relational and managerial capability • Might invoke issues around intellectual property	• Competing worldviews evoke conflicts around the "relevance" of knowledge • Potential subordinate role of social and cultural knowledge. • Broader impact limited	• Requires relevant networks and substantial investments • Skills to translate scientific knowledge into artefacts that drive consumer behaviour	• Engagement of relevant stakeholders • Reconciliation of conflicting practices and priorities of stakeholders

5.4 Conclusion and implications

Multidisciplinary approaches are associated with enhanced creativity and inventiveness, superior products, competitiveness, and positive effects on consumer behaviours and society (De Bernardi and Azucar, 2020; Rau et al., 2018). Yet, little is known about how these approaches allow NFFs to differentiate themselves and whether and how the conceptual distance between actors' disciplinary knowledge and practices affects these benefits. By offering an in-depth account of these approaches, using studies and extant research, this chapter sought to sensitise decision-makers to the approaches, benefits, and challenges that multidisciplinary endeavours in NFF firms entail.

By highlighting the potential pitfalls of narrow multidisciplinarity and the unreflective adoption of customer-centred methods like Design thinking, we urge firms to widen their innovation efforts beyond a small range of disciplines or stakeholders. This chapter thus complements calls to embrace Open Innovation in the nutraceutical sector (Siedlok et al., 2010). Beyond highlighting the value of multidisciplinary approaches for optimising product characteristics, we argue that broad multidisciplinary approaches can help firms shape their business context. As such, we empasise how innovations (especially radical ones) require both innovations in products and shaping of socio-economic contexts to generate long-term sustainable advantage and growth.

We also hope this chapter will prompt critical thinking and discussion about the role nutraceuticals play in society and how the sector is affected by and can respond to, broader socio-economic trends. The narrow definition of problems and solutions and the neglect of socio-cultural contexts fails to maximise the value generated by innovation in NFFs. In turn, we argue that a deeper integration of approaches, knowledge, skills, and tools from the Humanities and the Arts will help maximise the social, environmental, and economic benefits that are inherent to NFF products.

References

Almeida, F., de Paula, N., Pessali, H., 2014. Institutional entrepreneurship in building the Brazilian market of functional yogurts. British Food Journal 116 (1), 2–15. https://doi.org/10/f5n8pk.

Alongi, M., Anese, M., 2021. Re-thinking functional food development through a holistic approach. J. Funct. Foods 81, 104466. https://doi.org/10/gmmk3n.

Aventure. (2021). *Aventure.* Aventure. https://aventureab.com/. (Accessed 30 September 2021).

Bigliardi, B., Galati, F., 2013. Innovation trends in the food industry: the case of functional foods. Trends Food Sci. Technol. 31 (2), 118–129. https://doi.org/10/gf9zsp.

Bocken, N., Morales, L.S., Lehner, M., 2020. Sufficiency business strategies in the food industry—The case of Oatly. Sustainability 12 (3), 824. https://doi.org/10/ggtgkr.

Boehlje, M., Bröring, S., 2011. The increasing multifunctionality of agricultural raw materials: three dilemmas for innovation and adoption. International Food and Agribusiness Management Review 14 (2), 1–16.

Bogue, J., Collins, O., Troy, A.J., 2017. Market analysis and concept development of functional foods. In: Bagchi, D., Nair, S. (Eds.), Developing New Functional Food and Nutraceutical Products. Academic Press, pp. 29–45. https://doi.org/10.1016/B978-0-12-802780-6.00002-X.

Bröring, S., 2013. The role of open innovation in the industry convergence between foods and pharmaceuticals. In: Garcia Martinez, M. (Ed.), Open Innovation in the Food and Beverage Industry. Woodhead Publishing, Cambridge, UK, pp. 39–62. https://doi.org/10.1533/9780857097248.1.39.

Bröring, S., Cloutier, L.M., 2008. Value-creation in new product development within converging value chains: an analysis in the functional foods and nutraceutical industry. British Food Journal 110 (1), 76–97. https://doi.org/10/b4wsqg.

Bröring, S., Cloutier, L.M., Leker, J., 2006. The front end of innovation in an era of industry convergence: evidence from nutraceuticals and functional foods. R&D Management 36 (5), 487–498. https://doi.org/10/bfhf45.

Carlile, P.R., 2002. A pragmatic view of knowledge and boundaries: boundary objects in new product development. Organization Science 13 (4), 442–455.

Chiesa, V., Frattini, F., 2011. Commercializing technological innovation: learning from failures in high-tech markets*. Journal of Product Innovation Management 28 (4), 437–454. https://doi.org/10/b3z8vx.

Ciliberti, S., Carraresi, L., Bröring, S., 2016. Drivers of innovation in Italy: food versus pharmaceutical industry. British Food Journal 118 (6), 1292–1316. https://doi.org/10/f8ttrf.

De Bernardi, P., Azucar, D., De Bernardi, P., Azucar, D., 2020. The food system grand challenge: a climate smart and sustainable food system for a healthy europe. Innovation in Food Ecosystems: Entrepreneurship for a Sustainable Future. Springer International Publishing, Switzerland, pp. 1–25. https://doi.org/10.1007/978-3-030-33502-1_1.

Dell'Era, C. ;B, 2009. How can product semantics be embedded in product technologies? The case of the Italian wine industry. International Journal of Innovation Management 13, 411–439. https://doi.org/10/bxk6c7.

Evans, J., Terazono, E., 2021. The battle for the future of milk. Financial Times. https://www.ft.com/content/da70e996-a70b-484d-b3e6-ea8229253fc4. (Accessed 30 September 2021).

Fischer, A.R.H., Tobi, H., Ronteltap, A., 2011. When natural met social: a review of collaboration between the natural and social sciences. Interdisciplinary Science Reviews 36 (4), 341–358. https://doi.org/10.1179/030801811X13160755918688.

Foley, J.K., Michaux, K.D., Mudyahoto, B., Kyazike, L., Cherian, B., Kalejaiye, O., Ifeoma, O., Ilona, P., Reinberg, C., Mavindidze, D., Boy, E., 2021. Scaling up delivery of biofortified staple food crops globally: paths to nourishing millions. Food Nutr. Bull. 42 (1), 116–132. https://doi.org/10/gms4fm.

Frewer, L., Scholderer, J., Lambert, N., 2003. Consumer acceptance of functional foods: Issues for the future. British Food Journal 105 (10), 714–731. https://doi.org/10/c3bj6b.

Fuentes, C., Fuentes, M., 2017. Making a market for alternatives: marketing devices and the qualification of a vegan milk substitute. Journal of Marketing Management 33 (7–8), 529–555. https://doi.org/10/f99n5m.

Galati, F., Bigliardi, B., Petroni, A., 2016. Open innovation in food firms: implementation strategies, drivers and enabling factors. International Journal of Innovation Management 20 (03), 1650042. https://doi.org/10/gjmph5.

Gavetti, G., Helfat, C.E., Marengo, L., 2017. Searching, shaping, and the quest for superior performance. Strategy Science 2 (3), 194–209. https://doi.org/10/ghn4qw.

Hargrave, T.J., Van De Ven, A.H., 2006. A collective action model of institutional innovation. Acad. Manage. Rev. 31 (4), 864–888. https://doi.org/10/dq46nz.

Hartley, S., 2016. The fuzzy and the techie. Financial Times. https://www.ft.com/content/e25235dc-aa8a-11e6-9cb3-bb8207902122. (Accessed 17 January 2018).

Holm, P., Jarrick, A., Scott, D., 2015. Humanities World Report 2015. Palgrave Macmillan. 10.1057/9781137500281.

Huntington, H.P., 2000. Using traditional ecological knowledge in science: methods and applications. Ecol. Appl. 10 (5), 1270–1274. https://doi.org/10.1890/1051-0761(2000)010 [1270:UTEKIS]2.0.CO;2.

Huutoniemi, K., Klein, J.T., Bruun, H., Hukkinen, J., 2010. Analyzing interdisciplinarity: typology and indicators. Research Policy 39 (1), 79–88. https://doi.org/10/fg8jhp.

Ibert, O., Mueller, F.C., 2015. Network dynamics in constellations of cultural differences: relational distance in innovation processes in legal services and biotechnology. Research Policy 44 (1), 181–194. https://doi.org/10.1016/j.respol.2014.07.016.

Iskander, N., 2018. Design thinking is fundamentally conservative and preserves the status quo. Harv. Bus. Rev. https://hbr.org/2018/09/design-thinking-is-fundamentally-conservative-and-preserves-the-status-quo. (Accessed 26 June 2019).

Kalaitzandonakes, N., 2000. Functional foods: technical, institutional and market innovation. AgBioForum 3 (1), 2.

Khan, R.S., Grigor, J., Winger, R., Win, A., 2013. Functional food product development—opportunities and challenges for food manufacturers. Trends Food Sci. Technol. 30 (1), 27–37. https://doi.org/10/f4t6ts.

Klein, J.T., 2017. Typologies of Interdisciplinarity: The Boundary Work of Definition. In: Frodeman, R. (Ed.), The Oxford Handbook of Interdisciplinarity, 2nd ed. Oxford University Press, Oxford, UK, pp. 21–34.

Koch, C.H., 2020. Brands as activists: The Oatly case. Journal of Brand Management 27 (5), 593–606. https://doi.org/10/gh8hr5.

Kodama, M., Shibata, T., 2014. Strategy transformation through strategic innovation capability—a case study of Fanuc. R and D Management 44 (1), 75–103. https://doi.org/10.1111/radm.12041.

International. (2015). *Nutraceuticals:*. the future of intelligent food. Where food and pharmaceuticals converge. KPMG International. Available from: https://assets.kpmg/content/dam/kpmg/pdf/2015/04/neutraceuticals-the-future-of-intelligent-food.pdf. (Accessed 30 September 2021).

Liufu, J., Martirosyan, D., 2020. FFC's advancement of the establishment of functional food science. Functional Foods in Health and Disease 10 (8), 344–356.

Lowe, P., Phillipson, J., Wilkinson, K., 2013. Why social scientists should engage with natural scientists. Contemporary Social Science 8 (3), 207–222. https://doi.org/10/gdg3m7.

Mark-Herbert, C., 2004. Innovation of a new product category—Functional foods. Technovation 24 (9), 713–719. https://doi.org/10/c7wbmn.

Markides, C., 1997. Strategic innovation. Sloan Manage. Rev. 38 (3), 9–23.

Matthyssens, P., Vandenbempt, K., Berghman, L., 2008. Value innovation in the functional foods industry: deviations from the industry recipe. British Food Journal 110 (1), 144–155. https://doi.org/10/c2qbdd.

McGregor, S.L.T. (2015). Integral dispositions and transdisciplinary knowledge creation. http://integralleadershipreview.com/12548-115-integral-dispositions-transdisciplinary-knowledge-creation/. (Accessed 30 September 2021).

Oatly Group, AB. (2020). Oatly investors report. https://investors.oatly.com/static-files/4d70ce1e-ff99-4141-b943-30eb32215b98. (Accessed 18 September 2021).

Olmos-Penuela, J., Benneworth, P., Castro-Martinez, E., 2014. Are "STEM from Mars and SSH from Venus"? Challenging disciplinary stereotypes of research's social value. Science and Public Policy 41 (3), 384–400. https://doi.org/10/gdxrjw.

Pineda, S., 2017. HarvestPlus: A story of a nutrition revolution. Alliance Bioversity International. https://blog.ciat.cgiar.org/harvestplus-a-story-of-a-nutrition-revolution/. (Accessed 18 June 2021).

Rao, M., 2018. Sensemaking: Why human creativity and sensitivity are even more important in the age of AI. YourStory.Com. https://yourstory.com/2018/08/sensemaking-human-creativity-sensitivity-even-important-age-ai/. (Accessed 18 June 2021).

Rau, H., Goggins, G., Fahy, F., 2018. From invisibility to impact: Recognising the scientific and societal relevance of interdisciplinary sustainability research. Research Policy 47 (1), 266–276 Scopus. https://doi.org/10/gcs9q6.

Rhoten, D., 2004. Education: risks and rewards of an interdisciplinary research path. Science 306 (5704), 2046. https://doi.org/10/cb9pnn.

Ritvala, T., Granqvist, N., 2009. Institutional entrepreneurs and local embedding of global scientific ideas—the case of preventing heart disease in Finland. Scandinavian Journal of Management 25 (2), 133–145. https://doi.org/10/fdxsnh.

Sankaran, J.K., Mouly, V.S., 2007. Managing innovation in an emerging sector: the case of marine-based nutraceuticals. R&D Management 37 (4), 329–344. https://doi.org/10/dgm8fk.

Santini, A., Cammarata, S.M., Capone, G., Ianaro, A., Tenore, G.C., Pani, L., Novellino, E., 2018. Nutraceuticals: opening the debate for a regulatory framework. Br. J. Clin. Pharmacol. 84 (4), 659–672. https://doi.org/10/ggwztm.

Seidel, V.P., Fixson, S.K., 2013. Adopting design thinking in novice multidisciplinary teams: the application and limits of design methods and reflexive practices. Journal of Product Innovation Management 30 (1), 19–33. https://doi.org/10/gc7mdb.

Siedlok, F., Hibbert, P., 2014. The organization of interdisciplinary research: modes, drivers and barriers. International Journal of Management Reviews 16 (2), 194–210. https://doi.org/10/f5xwxw.

Siedlok, F., Smart, P., Gupta, A., 2010. Convergence and reorientation via open innovation: the emergence of nutraceuticals. Technology Analysis & Strategic Management 22 (5), 571–592. https://doi.org/10.1080/09537325.2010.488062.

Sijtsema, S.J., Fogliano, V., Hageman, M., 2020. Tool to support citizen participation and multidisciplinarity in food innovation: circular food design. Frontiers in Sustainable Food Systems 4, 582193. https://doi.org/10/gmmk3t.

Sreejith, S., 2021. AI in nutraceutical industry to enhance consumer experience. Accubits Blog. https://blog.accubits.com/ai-in-nutraceutical-industry-to-enhance-consumer-experience/. (Accessed 18 September 2021).

Szerszynski, B., Galarraga, M., 2013. Geoengineering knowledge: interdisciplinarity and the shaping of climate engineering research. Environment and Planning A: Economy and Space 45 (12), 2817–2824. https://doi.org/10.1068/a45647.

Talke, K., Salomo, S., Kock, A., 2011. Top management team diversity and strategic innovation orientation: the relationship and consequences for innovativeness and performance. Journal of Product Innovation Management 28 (6), 819–832. https://doi.org/10/bqz4ph.

Tkaczewska, J., Kulawik, P., Morawska-Tota, M., Zając, M., Guzik, P., Tota, Ł., Pająk, P., Duliński, R., Florkiewicz, A., Migdał, W., 2021. Protocol for designing new functional food with the addition of food industry by-products, using design thinking techniques—a case study of a snack with antioxidant properties for physically active people. Foods 10 (4), 694. https://doi.org/10/gmqhr3.

Tripsas, M., Gavetti, G., 2000. Capabilities, cognition, and inertia: evidence from digital imaging. Strategic Management Journal 21 (10/11), 1147–1161. JSTOR. https://doi.org/10.1002/1097-0266(200010/11)21:10/11<1147::AID-SMJ128>3.0.CO;2-R.

Tumilowicz, A., Neufeld, L.M., Pelto, G.H., 2016. Using ethnography in implementation research to improve nutrition interventions in populations. Maternal & Child Nutrition 11 (Suppl 3), 55–72. https://doi.org/10/f79fmx.

van Kleef, E., van Trijp, H.C.M., Luning, P., Jongen, W.M.F., 2002. Consumer-oriented functional food development: How well do functional disciplines reflect the 'voice of the consumer'? Trends Food Sci. Technol. 13 (3), 93–101. https://doi.org/10/c975r3.

Wierzbicka, A., 2011. Defining 'the humanities'. Culture & Psychology 17 (1), 31–46. https://doi.org/10/bjpmrw.

SECTION 2

Strategy

CHAPTER 6

Nutraceutical and functional value of carob-based products
The LBG Sicilia Srl Case Study

Mario Testa[a], Ornella Malandrino[a], Cristina Santini[b], Stefania Supino[b]
[a]DISA-MIS, University of Salerno, Fisciano, SA, Italy
[b]University San Raffaele Rome, Italy

6.1 Introduction

The rediscovery and use of ancient plants that have best adapted to their growth territory are crucial to preserving biodiversity and promoting sustainable agricultural practices. The research community and drug and food industries have focused the last few years on the full exploitation of natural products to discover new pharmaceutical targets with promising potential and the enrichment of various food products with high biological-value natural substances. Various food products based on the bioactivities of plant compounds have also been developed to maintain health, prevent disease, and enhance overall health and well-being.

Moreover, with rising health consciousness, consumers have been gradually shifting toward healthy food, and the growing trend of plant-based foods is driving the market. Among the species cultivated since ancient times and neglected for many decades, the carob (*Ceratonia siliqua*) is enjoying renewed interest owing to the valuable applications of its derivatives—principally of locust bean gum (LBG), used as a food stabilizer, thickening agent, and emulsifier (E410). In addition, it is used for pharmaceutical, medical, nutraceutical, and functional purposes.

The carob tree requires limited rainfall and it is sustainable cultivation. In this scenario, the carob plays a central role in human health benefits, the economy, and the environment.

This chapter aims to review and highlight the beneficial aspects of carob fruit and its potential for use as a functional and nutraceutical ingredient in the food industry, opening new perspectives for this sustainable crop. Furthermore, the chapter describes the case study of LGB Sicilia

Srl, which aims to underline the opportunities to improve and optimize the production chain of sustainable natural resources, such as the carob, increasingly requested by the global agro-industrial market. Investments in soft technologies, vertical integration, lean organization, and high-quality natural products have made the success of this company feasible worldwide, creating a mix of values and distinctive characteristics, among which flexibility and sustainability emerge strongly.

6.2 Nutritional and functional value of carob-based products

The carob is an evergreen tree cultivated in Mediterranean countries, such as Portugal, Italy, Spain, Morocco, Greece (Durazzo et al., 2014) and, more recently, in other areas such as California, Arizona, Mexico, Chile, Argentina, Australia, South Africa, and India (Battle & Tous, 1997). It is a common belief that from the word carob comes "carat", a unit of weight of gold and precious stones, as the carob seeds were used in ancient times for weighing. It is a wild tree, resistant to fire, exploiting barren soil unsuitable for other crops (marginal soil) and protecting them from corrosion. It is resistant to adversity and the main pathologies. According to some studies, carob species are recommended to reforest degraded areas threatened by desertification and disadvantaged rural areas (Gharnit & Ennabili, 2016; Vekiari et al., 2011).

The carob tree has shallow rainfall requirements and can be developed with minimal or no irrigation. This tree can improve soil fertility by fixing nitrogen and carbon dioxide three times more than other woody crops (Cordis, European Commission, 2018). It can live up to 300 years and can exceed 15 m in height. Its average productivity varies between 90 and 115 kg/year, and it may increase up to double that amount, depending on climate and soil conditions (Ghrabi, 2005).

The traditional carob fruit (pods) of cultivated varieties generally contains two major parts: the pulp (90%) and the seeds (10%). The seed consists of germ, endosperm, and husk. Because the germ and the endosperm are used in different (food and/or nonfood) applications, it is also necessary to separate the different seed fractions (Fig. 6.1).

The chemical composition of the pulp depends on the cultivar, origin, and harvesting time. Carob pulp is high (48%–56%) in total sugar content (mainly sucrose, glucose, and fructose) and holds about 18% cellulose and hemicelluloses and relatively low content of fats and protein (Stavrou et al., 2018). Because of the high sugar content, the pulp is used to make syrups, molasses, or flour used as a cocoa substitute since it has no caffeine

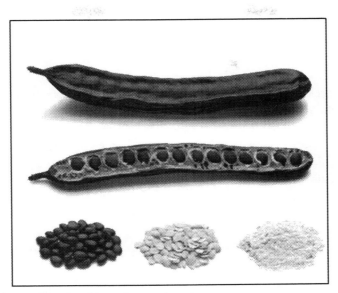

Fig. 6.1 The carob pod and its main constituents.

theobromine but has a low fat content (Loullis & Pinakoulaki, 2018; Aydin & Özdemir, 2017; Biner et al., 2007; Yousif & Alghzawi, 2000; Calixto & Cañellas, 1982).

Ripe carob pods also contain condensed tannins (16%–20% of dry weight) (Wursch et al., 1984). Minerals such as calcium, phosphorus, potassium, magnesium, sodium, and iron are present, proposing carob pods as an alternative source of minerals (Ayaz et al., 2007; Papaefsthatiou et al., 2018). Ripe carob pods also contain many polyphenols (Avallone et al., 1997; Bravo et al., 1994, Marakis, 1996; Makris et al., 2004; Stavrou et al., 2018). The main categories of phenolic compounds found in carob fruit are phenolic acids, gallotannins, and flavonoids (Goulas et al., 2016).

Among the different carob products (husk, endosperm, germ, and pulp), the economic importance of carob pod comes from the industrial utilization of locust bean gum (LBG), an authorized food additive in the European Union, as E410 (European Food Safety Authority [EFSA], 2017). LBG comes from the seed's endosperm. From the chemical point of view, LBG is a galactomannan, a versatile hydrocolloid used as a stiffener and stabilizer of emulsions in food industries and textile, pharmaceutical, or biomedical sectors. On the other hand, the pulp is considered a by-product of the carob pod industry. It represents an important source of nutrients, such as carbohydrates (mainly sugars and fibre), minerals, amino acids, and vitamins, among other components. Due to the characteristics mentioned, carob pulp has been used as a cheap source for animal nutrition and humans in times of famine.

Other relevant components in carob pulp are the secondary metabolites, such as phenolic acids, flavonoids, and tannins. They have functional properties and provide health benefits (e.g., antioxidant, anti-inflammatory, and anti-ageing properties) to the human body (Rodríguez-Solana et al., 2021). Fig. 6.2 summarizes the main chemical constituents in carob pulp and seed with nutritional and health-promoting properties.

Many studies have shown that carobs and their products can promote human health and help prevent specific chronic diseases (Papaefstathiou et al., 2018). In particular, they have antiproliferative and apoptotic activity against cancer cells, help treat diarrhoea symptoms, and present antihyperlipidemia and antidiabetic properties due to high antioxidants, polyphenols, and high fibre content effects (Theophilou et al., 2017). Therefore, they are considered an ideal food for diabetes (Youssef et al., 2013). Carob flour (from carob seeds) is used to manufacture dietetic products and products for celiac patients (gluten-free products) (Tsatsaragkou et al., 2014).

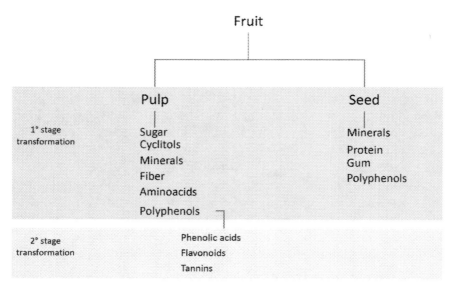

Adapted from Goulas et al., 2016

Fig. 6.2 Major constituents in carob fruit with nutritional and health-promoting properties (adapted from Goulas et al., 2016).

6.3 The Market

Over time, the world production of carob has decreased considerably. Currently, it is around 187 kt; Portugal (42 kt), Italy (37 kt), and Spain (23 kt) represent 55% of this production. Over the past decades, Italian carob production has decreased significantly: from 76 kt in 1970 to about 25 kt in 2010 and around 29 kt in 2018 (FAOSTAT, 2020). The main geographical areas of production in Italy are in Sicily (36 kt) and Puglia (0,6 kt). Sicily contributes to national production with 97% and world production with a share equal to 19%. The cultivation, production, marketing, and transformation of carob mainly occurs in the Sicilian provinces of Ragusa and Syracuse. All Italian production is addressed to the domestic market. Seeds are separated from pods using a process known as *kibbling* (Pegg, 2012). Pods are broken between two rollers and seeds separated from the rest of the pods using special screens. Acid and heat (chemical peeling), or heat and mechanical abrasion, help to remove the hull. These processes also facilitate germ separation from the endosperm, which is then ground and graded by particle size and viscosity and sold as LBG. The pulp can be used for livestock feed and human consumption. After roasting, the pulp can be employed by the confectionery industry as a substitute for cocoa (cacao), in the production of dietary foods, for example, "gluten-free", or nutraceuticals. LBG consists chiefly of high-molecular-weight hydrocolloidal polysaccharides (galactomannans), composed of galactose and mannose units, a substance capable of absorbing water up to 40 times its dry weight. The Italian production of carob flour is about 5,5 kt, all produced in Sicily.

The world volume size of the LBG market is approximately 12 kt/ year, predominantly for ice cream and cheese applications. Unilever, Nestle, and Kraft are heavy users. According to some forecasts, the LBG market was valued at 103 million USD in 2020, and it is expected to reach 121.9 million USD by the end of 2026, growing at a Compounded Average Growth Rate (CAGR) of 2.4% (WBC, 2020). The Italian share of the international market is about 46% (47 million USD). The LBG world market has increased in terms of request and, then, in terms of price. The growing concern about the availability of LBG due to shortages of the raw material and the continuing solid demand based on its excellent image as a 'natural' food is causing an increase in price. According to modern market needs and progressions, the importance of carob is expected to grow globally due to the trend toward health and nutrient supplements, the need for biological and gluten-free products, and the need for natural hydrocolloids (Papaefstathiou et al., 2018).

6.4 The role of consumers' final preferences

Carob progressively became a strategic input for the food industry. According to the type of food product, companies have to identify inputs' features that better address consumers' expectations. Background research describes cases and examples in different contexts and situations. Thus, the nutritional properties of carob, together with its enormous versatility as an input for the food industry, represent a research theme that has progressively attracted scholars from different fields.

Aydin and Özdemir (2017) outline the steps to develop carob flour–based functional spread in nutrition snacks for children. The authors outline the relevant attributes for consumers. It emerges, for example, that spreadability is a key textural attribute that affects consumer acceptance of confectionary—or gelled—products. According to the study, particle size influences spreadability. As a consequence, food producers' suppliers should consider consumers' final preferences when planning their production processes.

Other studies on consumers' preferences in bakery production: Issaoui et al. (2021) have outlined the importance of integrating consumer testings in developing carob-based flours to produce bakery products. Colour, texture, aroma, flavour, and taste are essential for consumers. In addition to the final results of tests and hedonic evaluation, what emerges from the study is the relevance of carob for industry and bakeries, which have to search for multiple alternatives to traditional products to face the diffuse gluten intolerance among consumers. Furthermore, the study outlines the role of the production process in modifying initial input properties. This is, of course, not new to food technologies. However, it is an issue to highlight since this situation can influence carob-based input suppliers.

Other studies are available that show the versatility of the input: research ranges from yoghurt (Aydinol et al., 2021), cookies (Babiker et al., 2020), alternative milk (Srour et al., 2016), and pasta (Altiner & Hallaç, 2020) to the pharmaceutical industry in general (Dionìsio et Grenha, 2012). The research shows that the wide range of possibilities for carob suggests that suppliers pay close attention to what is relevant for consumers.

The literature shows the benefits for those companies that shape their strategic planning, assuming market orientation as one of the pillars of their managerial mindset (see, among the others, the work by Lingreen et al., 2010). In general, having a solid market orientation can help reduce market failure. For those who supply inputs for multiple and diversified usages in product processes, being market oriented means acquiring competencies and knowledge about final product features and needs that emerge from different customers.

6.5 Case Study: LBG Sicilia Srl

6.5.1 Overview and core business

In Italy, LGB Sicilia Srl is currently the second largest LGB producer globally, after DuPont. Founded in 2001, LBG Sicilia Srl has become one of the leading companies in the world market, supplying the largest food companies in more than 90 countries.

The start of this interesting Italian enterprise dates back to the 1950s, thanks to Rosario Licitra, father of the current owner of the company LBG Sicilia Srl, Giancarlo Licitra. Its activity consisted of the storage and marketing of carob pods, grown in the Ragusa area and its surroundings (Sicily), an area included in the UNESCO World Heritage List since 2002, where about 95% of the raw material currently processed is still produced today at the plant in Ragusa. The rest (5%) of the processed raw material comes from Puglia.

The Carrube Kibbling Flora company was established in Ragusa, with products sold to customers located in Ragusa.

LBG was founded in 2001 with an innovative plant in the industrial area of Ragusa, and the activities were expanded to Functional Systems and Contract Blending Service Business (2013). A new planned expansion in 2021 aimed to double production, storage capacity, and laboratory operations to increase production volume and the range of products (including pectins and proteins) offered to international markets.

The idea that led to the company's current success dates back to 2001, with Giancarlo Licitra. Giancarlo Licitra, who holds a degree in Business Administration from the University of Catania (1988), knowledge of the English language acquired at the Business School, University of Edinburgh, received the honour of Cavaliere del Lavoro in May 2018 from the President of the Italian Republic, Sergio Mattarella. Indeed, with the adoption of a profound diversification strategy (Table 6.1), he has changed the core business of the family enterprise. The company shifted from the marketing of raw materials to the vertical integration (Fig. 6.3) of all phases, from agricultural and trade to manufacturing, transformation, blending, and sale of derivatives worldwide. Among the company's various clients, we can find several multinational customers, such as Nestlé, Lactalis, Muller, Cargill, Mars, and others.

In a few years, with its SEEDGUM® range, it has become one of the leading companies in the worldwide LBG market, supplying the most relevant food companies, as noted earlier. In 2013, continuing its vertical

Table 6.1 LBG Products

Texture Ingredients	Plant Based Proteins
Locust bean gum	Carob proteins
Locust bean gum pet food	Plant-based proteins
Standardized pectins	Functional proteins
Texture Ingredients Systems	**Vegetable Fibers**
Dairy systems	Carob seed fibers
Ice cream systems	Vegetable fibers
Fruit-based systems	Functional fibers systems
Pet food systems	**Animal Nutrition**
Convenience systems	Sugars
	Fibers

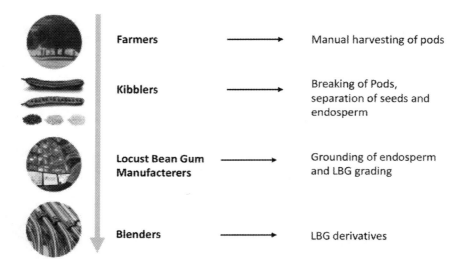

Fig. 6.3 Vertical integration.

integration strategy, the company completed a significant investment. The company created two new divisions: (1) SOLMIX®: Design, Production and Marketing of Stabilizing and Texturant Systems, with particular attention to LBG-based systems; and (2) BLENDTECH®: Superior Quality Standard for Contract Blending Service.

LBG Sicilia Srl has always been committed to enhancing its products through targeted quality controls and production processes characterized by highly innovative technologies. The processing plant, also characterized by the innovative open-space structure in the Ragusa industrial area, employs about 40 people. The production capacity is 10 kt of fresh product transformed into 9 kt of kibbled pulp and 1 kt of seeds.

Current production is 3550 t/year for food and 1500 t/year for pet food, with around 8 million euros annual turnover. The present organization of the company is the result of an efficient and cost-effective vertical integration of all phases of the supply chain.

The company has established a direct and collaborative relationship with farmers. They have avoided intermediation and promoted the cultivation of carob trees: a surface of more than 35 hectares and 5000 carob trees was planted in 1998, then grafted in 2008 with different cultivars. Following this policy allowed the company to achieve upstream direct control of the quality of the raw material. At the same time, downstream, the company aimed to pursue customer satisfaction on the world market and improve by-products (over 99%) to reduce the impact of waste. The company fully integrates a circular-economy paradigm by minimizing the negative environmental consequences of productive activities and, overall, creating value.

Constant technological innovation aimed at achieving food safety, quality control, sustainability, and flexibility characterize the manufacturing and transformation stages approach. LBG's commitment strategically employs certifications (Fig. 6.4) to support its goals: Iso 22000 (Food Safety Management System), Organic (certification looking at all aspects of organic manufacturing and production, storage, and sales), Sedex Membership (Empowering Responsible Supply Chain), BRCGS (Food Safety Certification), Kosher (certification in order to assure consumers that all ingredients, derivatives, tools, and machinery comply with a strict policy of kosher food laws, including

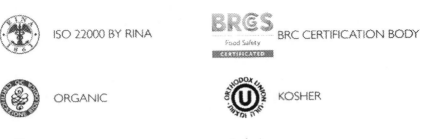

Fig. 6.4 Some quality certifications.

cleanliness, purity and quality), Halal (certification of products in compliance with the precepts of Islamic law), and Ecovadis (Silver Sustainability Rating). Moreover, LBG Sicilia is achieving Iso 14001 (Environmental Management Systems) and 45001 (Occupational Health and Safety Management Systems) certifications. It is also publishing the first Certified Sustainability Annual Report. With the report's publication, the company aims to show its stakeholders the commitment to sustainability understood by its three main pillars: economic, environmental, and social dimensions.

6.5.2 Values, strategies, and perspectives

LBG Sicilia Srl is a private and independent company founded in 2001, specializing in high-quality functional ingredients and systems for the food industry. Innovation is the keyword for understanding its success: since its beginnings, the company has focused its investments on advancing every manufacturing process feature, as highlighted in this section. The results achieved mainly derive from imperatives that the company has incorporated into its values: vertical integration, improvement in technologies, food safety, organization and flexibility, and—last, but not least—sustainability.

Vertical integration. The company's strategy has always been based on vertical integration to obtain synergies and competitive advantages in the supply chain, joint production technologies, and final markets. The company has in-depth knowledge of the whole process: starting from carob pod production, through carob kibbling, locust bean gum production, and functional systems based on LBG, such as ice cream stabilizers or sauce texturing systems.

Technologies. LBG Sicilia believes in standardization, lower production costs, and higher quality by reducing cross-contamination risks by adopting a pushed automation.

Food safety. Chemical-free LBG production and the revolutionary Blendtech Blending Plant upgrade the usual standards to pharma ones. The automated management allows cross-contamination prevention and improved traceability guarantees contamination-free processes. Moreover, the company has always believed that naturalness is the future of the food industry.

Organization and flexibility. The company has an efficient structure due to approaches that range from lean production to the Industry 4.0 paradigm. The vast network of relationships that the company has established in more than 90 countries globally and dealing with different needs and regulations systems drive the enormous efforts undertaken by the company.

Sustainability. This is a commitment that is pursued through different approaches. The cultivation of carob trees does not require fertilizers, pesticides, or even irrigation. This allows the natural environment to absorb greenhouse gas (GHGs) emissions while preventing hydrogeological instability. Furthermore, the carob seeds are dehusked only by multistage thermo-mechanical treatments; consequently, the process is chemical-free. Moreover, the lack of chemicals allows the correct recycling of almost all waste through the valorization of products sold for different applications. The energy used comes from renewable sources and precisely from photovoltaic panels.

Innovation in manufacturing technology, smart commercial approach, food safety improvement, and in-depth knowledge of international laws are only some of the reasons for LBG Sicilia Srl's success. Its real secret is passion and a unique family spirit of dedication and great flexibility, unusual for an international company.

Its customers in more than 90 countries worldwide say that LBG Sicilia Srl functional ingredients and blends are noteworthy for the reliability, flexibility, and commitment that this company puts into every ounce of product. LBG Sicilia Srl is proud of their satisfaction and of being part of the everyday life of millions of people throughout the world with their successful products.

Excellence is often the consequence of a particular attitude regarding work resulting from a unique mix of values and distinction points leading to very specific recipes and outstanding outcomes, both in strategy and competitiveness.

6.6 Conclusions

In recent years, healthy foods and lifestyles in the pursuit of health promotion and disease prevention have become popular. The high dietary fibre content of carob, its bioactive compounds, and beneficial effects make this input an ideal ingredient for developing novel healthy food products. Incorporating carob fruit and its derivative products in food formulations enhances nutritional and functional value. In particular, they show antiproliferative and apoptotic activity against cancer cells. They are suggested for diarrhoea symptoms and have antihyperlipidemia and antidiabetic effects due to their high antioxidants, polyphenols, and fibre content. Therefore, this type of food is ideal for people with diabetes. Carob flour (from carob seeds) is used for dietetic products and products for celiac patients (gluten-free products).

The rediscovery and use of ancient plants adapted to their growth territory are crucial to preserving biodiversity and promoting sustainable agricultural practices from a bioeconomy perspective. The carob tree is just one of the several opportunities in this direction. Such an approach should unite all actors across territories, promoting resource-efficient value chains.

It will require addressing the systemic challenges that cut across the different sectors, including synergies and trade-offs, to facilitate the deployment of a long-term vision of the pathways needed to enhance bioeconomy models. Although the multiple applications suggested by the bioeconomy and circular economy to overcome the challenge of transforming the food system towards sustainable paradigms are still in the early phase, the market success of LBG Sicilia demonstrates the relevance of investing in this business area. Ensuring food security and safety constitutes one of the most significant future challenges. At the same time, it represents an unequalled opportunity and a key tool to tackle these very complex challenges and can lead to sustainable economic growth.

The market success of LGB Sicilia highlights the opportunities to improve and optimize the production chain of sustainable natural resources, such as the carob, increasingly requested by the world agro-industrial market.

The described case shows the versatility of carob, and it opens many questions about the managerial implication of such a product. There is no doubt that carob has growing market potential, and it has high margins and different end markets due to its multiple employment in the food industry. Therefore, as we have previously outlined, acquiring information about how inputs interact with production processes is relevant. The chapter highlights that having market orientation means gaining information about the consumer's final preference to modify input features and meet users' final expectations. A similar scenario implies that companies improve their knowledge and information: it becomes relevant to know what directs customers' preferences and the needs and preferences that emerge from consumers. In this perspective, consumer science tools can provide valuable information for understanding the appraisal of product features. Therefore, companies that operate as suppliers in the food supply chain, such as LGB, in the future can cooperate with their customers to carry out research to measure and evaluate consumers' ultimate preferences.

References

Altiner, D.D., Hallaç, Ş., 2020. The effect of soy flour and carob flour addition on the physicochemical, quality, and sensory properties of pasta formulations. Int. J. Agric. Environ. Food Sci. 4 (4), 406–417.

Avallone, R., Plessi, M., Baraldi, M., Monzani, A., 1997. Determination of chemical composition of carob (Ceratonia siliqua): protein, fat, carbohydrates, and tannins. J. Food Compos. Anal. 10 (2), 166–172.

Ayaz, F.A., Torun, H., Ayaz, S., Correia, P.J., Alaiz, M., Sanz, C., Strnad, M., 2007. Determination of chemical composition of anatolian carob pod (Ceratonia siliqual.): sugars, amino and organic acids, minerals and phenolic compounds. J. Food Qual. 30 (6), 1040–1055.

Aydın, S., Özdemir, Y., 2017. Development and characterization of carob flour based functional spread for increasing use as nutritious snack for children. J. Food Qual., 1–7.

Aydinol Sonmez, P., Ozcan, T., 2021. Assessment of structure and sensory characteristics of reduced fat yoghurt manufactured with carob bean gum polysaccharides. Food Sci. Technol. 42.

Babiker, E.E., Özcan, M.M., Ghafoor, K., Al Juhaimi, F., Ahmed, I.A.M., Almusallam, I.A., 2020. Physico-chemical and bioactive properties, fatty acids, phenolic compounds, mineral contents, and sensory properties of cookies enriched with carob flour. J. Food Process. Preserv. 44 (10), e14745.

Battle, I., Tous, J., 1997. Carob tree: Ceratonia siliqua L. – Promoting the conservation and use of underutilized and neglected crops, 17. Institute of Plant Genetics and Crop Plant Research. Rome: Gatersleben/International Plant Genetic Resources Institute.

Biner, B., Gubbuk, H., Karhan, M., Aksu, M., Pekmezci, M., 2007. Sugar profiles of the pods of cultivated and wild types of carob bean in Turkey. Food Chem. 100 (4), 1453–1455.

Bravo, L., Grados, N., Saura-Calixto, F., 1994. Composition and potential uses of mesquite pods (Prosopis pallida L.): comparison with carob pods (Ceratonia siliqua L.). J. Sci. Food Agric. 65, 303–306.

Calixto, F.S., Cañellas, J., 1982. Components of nutritional interest in carob pods (Ceratonia siliqua). J. Sci. Food Agric. 33 (12), 1319–1323.

Cordis, European Commission. Valorization of the carob pod into an added value natural extract for the food and drink industry, (2018) https://cordis.europa.eu/project/id/790025/it.

Durazzo, A., Turfani, V., Narducci, V., Azzini, E., Maiani, G., Carcea, M., 2014. Nutritional characterisation and bioactive components of commercial carobs flours. Food Chem. 153, 109–113.

EFSA, Mortensen, A., Aguilar, F., Crebelli, R., Di Domenico, A., Frutos, M. J., Dusemund, B., 2017. Re-evaluation of locust bean gum (E 410) as a food additive. Efsa Journal 15 (1), https://doi.org/10.2903/j.efsa.2017.4646.

FAOSTAT, (2020) *Food and Agriculture Organization of the United Nations, Final Data.* http://www.fao.org/faostat/en/#data/QC.

Gharnit, N., Ennabili, A., 2016. Categories of carob tree (*Ceratonia siliqua* L.) from Morocco. Int. J. Fruit Sci. 16 (3), 259–274.

Ghrabi, Z., 2005. A Guide to Medicinal Plants in North Africa. IUCN Centre For Mediterranean Cooperation Published, Malaga, Spain, pp. 79–81.

Goulas, V., Stylos, E., Chatziathanasiadou, M.V., Mavromoustakos, T., Tzakos Andreas, G., 2016. Functional components of carob fruit: linking the chemical and biological space international. Int. J. Mol. Sci, 171875. doi:10.3390/ijms17111875.

Issaoui, M., Flamini, G., Delgado, A., 2021. Sustainability opportunities for Mediterranean food products through new formulations based on carob flour (Ceratonia siliqua L.). Sustainability 13 (14), 8026.

Lingreen, A., Hingley, M., Custance, P., 2010. *Market orientation: Transforming food and agribusiness around the customer.* Routledge. Gower Publishing.

Loullis, A., Pinakoulaki, E., 2018. Carob as cocoa substitute: a review on composition, health benefits and food applications. Eur. Food Res. Technol. 244, 959–977.

Makris, D.P., Kefalas, P., 2004. Carob pods (*Ceratonia siliqua* L.) as a source of polyphenolic antioxidants. Food Technol. Biotechnol. 42, 105–108.

Marakis, S., 1996. Carob bean in food and feed: current status and future potentials—a critical appraisal. J. Food Sci. Technol. 33, 365–383.

Papaefstathiou, E., Agapiou, A., Giannopoulos, S., Kokkinofta, R., 2018. Nutritional characterization of carobs and traditional carob products. Food Sci. Nutr. https://doi.org/10.1002/fsn3.776.

Pegg, A.M., 2012. The application of natural hydrocolloids to foods and beverages. Natural food additives, ingredients and flavourings. Woodhead Publishing, pp. 175–196.

Rodríguez-Solana, R., Romano, A., Moreno-Rojas, J.M., 2021. Carob pulp: A nutritional and functional by-product worldwide spread in the formulation of different food products and beverages. A review. Processes 9 (7), 1146.

Srour, N., Daroub, H., Toufeili, I., Olabi, A., 2016. Developing a carob-based milk beverage using different varieties of carob pods and two roasting treatments and assessing their effect on quality characteristics. J. Sci. Food Agric. 96 (9), 3047–3057.

Stavrou, I.J., Christou, A., Kapnissi-Christodoulou, C.P., 2018. Polyphenols in carobs: A review on their composition, antioxidant capacity and cytotoxic effects, and health impact. Food Chem. 269, 355–374.

Theophilou, I.C., Neophytou, C.M., Constantinou, A.I., 2017. Carob and its components in the management of gastrointestinal disorders. J. Hepatol. Gastroenterol 1 (005).

Tsatsaragkou, K., Gounaropoulos, G., Mandala, I., 2014. Development of gluten free bread containing carob flour and resistant starch. LWT-Food Sci. Technol. 58 (1), 124–129.

Vekiari, S.A., Ouzounidou, G., Ozturk, M., Görk, G., 2011. Variation of quality characteristics in Greek and Turkish carob pods during fruit development. Proc. Soc. Behav. Sci. 19, 750–755.

WBC, (2020) Locust bean gum (E-410) market 2020 global industry brief analysis by top countries data with market size is expected to see growth of 121.9 million USD till 2026. http://www.wboc.com/story/42437083/locust-bean-gum-e-410-market-2020-global-industry-brief-analysis-by-top-countries-data-with-market-size-is-expected-to-see-growth-of-1219-million-usd.

Wursch, P., Delvedovo, S., Rosset, J., Smiley, M., 1984. The tannin granules from ripe carob pod. Lebensm. Wiss. Technol 17, 351–354.

Youssef, M.K.E., El-Manfaloty, M.M., Ali, H.M., 2013. Assessment of proximate chemical composition, nutritional status, fatty acid composition and phenolic compounds of carob (Ceratonia siliqua L.). Food and Public Health 3 (6), 304–308.

Yousif, A.K., Alghzawi, H.M., 2000. Processing and characterization of carob powder. Food Chem. 69 (3), 283–287.

CHAPTER 7

Breaking the cycle of malnutrition through sustainable business models: The case of ready-to-use therapeutic foods

Mario Testa[a], Francesco Polese[a], Sergio Barile[b]
[a]DISA-MIS, University of Salerno, Fisciano, SA, Italy
[b]Sapienza University, Rome, Italy

7.1 Introduction

The FAO Agricultural Development Economics Division in collaboration with the Statistics Division of the Economic and Social Development Department and a team of technical experts from FAO, IFAD, UNICEF, WFP, and WHO, in the report "State of Food Security and Nutrition in the World 2019. Safeguarding against economic slowdowns and downturns" (FAO, IFAD, UNICEF, WFP and WHO, Rome 2019)[a] highlights that safeguard food security and nutrition is a critical issue in order to already have in place economic and social policies to counteract the effects of adverse economic cycles. In the longer term, nevertheless, this will only be achievable through promotion pro-poor and inclusive structural conversion, particularly in countries that rely deeply on trade in primary commodities. Economic shocks are contributing to prolonging and worsening the harshness of food crises caused mainly by conflict and climate shocks. Economic slowdowns or downturns undermine food security and nutrition where inequalities are greater. Income and wealth inequality

---

[a]The State of Food Security and Nutrition in the World is an annual flagship report jointly prepared by FAO, IFAD, UNICEF, WFP, and WHO to inform on progress towards ending hunger, achieving food security, and improving nutrition and to provide in depth analysis on key challenges for achieving this goal in the context of the 2030 Agenda for Sustainable Development. The report targets a wide audience, including policy-makers, international organizations, academic institutions, and the general public.

Case Studies on the Business of Nutraceuticals, Functional and Super Foods
DOI: https://doi.org/10.1016/B978-0-12-821408-4.00001-8
121

are strongly associated with undernutrition and amplify the likelihood of severe food insecurity, principally for low-income countries, compared with middle-income countries. The FAO report tracks world hunger using the prevalence of undernourishment (PoU), one of the global Sustainable Development Goals (SDGs) monitoring framework indicators[b] (SDG Target 2.1), as well as using the prevalence of moderate or severe food insecurity (SDG Target 2.2) based on the Food Insecurity Experience Scale. The 2030 Agenda, indeed, underlines that food insecurity is more than hunger. The Zero Hunger goal aims not simply to "eradicate hunger", but also to "ensure access by all people [...] to safe, nutritious and sufficient food all year round" (SDG Target 2.1) and to "eradicate all forms of malnutrition" (SDG Target 2.2). The COVID-19 pandemic is intensifying the vulnerabilities and inadequacies of global food systems and of all the activities and processes affecting the production, distribution, and consumption of food so that this circumstance further questions the achievement of the goal Zero Hunger. Among the aims of the SDG 2 Targets, it emerges that by 2030 it is necessary to double the agricultural productivity and incomes of small-scale food producers, in particular women, indigenous peoples, family farmers, pastoralists, and fishers, including through secure and equal access to land, other productive resources, and inputs, knowledge, financial services, markets and opportunities for value addition and nonfarm employment.[c]

[b]"The 2030 Agenda for Sustainable Development, adopted by all United Nations Member States in 2015, provides a shared blueprint for peace and prosperity for people and the planet, now and into the future. "At its heart are the 17 Sustainable Development Goals (SDGs), which are an urgent call for action by all countries - developed and developing - in a global partnership. They recognize that ending poverty and other deprivations must go hand-in-hand with strategies that improve health and education, reduce inequality, and spur economic growth – all while tackling climate change and working to preserve our oceans and forests". See, https://sdgs.un.org/goals. Sustainable Development Goal 2 is Zero Hunger: by 2030 end hunger and ensure access by all people, in particular the poor and people in vulnerable situations, including infants, to safe, nutritious and sufficient food all year round, end all forms of malnutrition, including achieving, by 2025, the internationally agreed targets on stunting and wasting in children under 5 years of age, and address the nutritional needs of adolescent girls, pregnant and lactating women and older persons and achieve food security and improved nutrition and promote sustainable agriculture.

[c]See, https://www.undp.org/content/undp/en/home/sustainable-development-goals/goal-2-zerohunger/targets.html.

7.2 The state of the art on food security and nutrition in the world: A summary

The data explained in the relevant report "The State of Food Security and Nutrition in the World. Transforming Food Systems for Affordable Healthy" (FAO, IFAD, UNICEF, WFP and WHO, Rome 2020) reveals that the world is not on track to achieve the SDG 2.1 and SDG 2.2 Zero Hunger target by 2030. If recent trends continue, the number of people affected by hunger would increase further. A preliminary assessment suggests that the COVID-19 pandemic may add between 83 and 132 million people to the total number of undernourished in the world in 2020 depending on the economic growth scenario.[d] The reasons for the increase are multiple. Much of the recent increase in food insecurity can be attributed to the greater number of conflicts, often exacerbated by climate-related shocks. Even in some peaceful settings, food security has deteriorated as a result of economic slowdowns threatening access to food for the poor. Food insecurity can worsen diet quality and consequently increase the risk of various forms of malnutrition, potentially leading to undernutrition.

Combined projections of recent trends in the size and composition of the population, in the total food availability, and in the degree of inequality in food access point to an increase of the PoU by almost 1%. As a result, the global number of undernourished people in 2030 would exceed 840 million, not considering the potential impact of the COVID-19 pandemic (Fig. 7.1).

The PoU in Africa was 19.1% of the population in 2019, or more than 250 million undernourished people, up from 17.6% in 2014. This prevalence is more than twice the world average (8.9%) and is the highest among all regions.

Asia is home to more than half of the total undernourished people in the world, an estimated 381 million people in 2019. Yet, the PoU in the population for the region is 8.3%, below the world average (8.9%), and less than half of that of Africa. Asia has shown progress in reducing the number of hungry people in recent years, down by 8 million since 2015. In Latin America and the Caribbean, the PoU was 7.4% in 2019, below the world prevalence of 8.9%, which still translates into almost 48 million undernourished people. The region has seen a rise in hunger in the past few years, with the number of undernourished people increasing by 9 million

[d]See, https://www.who.int/news/item/13-07-2020-as-more-go-hungry-and-malnutrition-persists-achieving-zero-hunger-by-2030-in-doubt-un-report-warns.

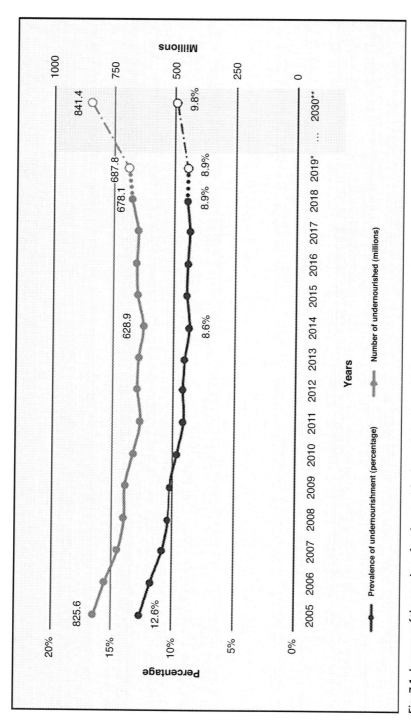

Fig. 7.1 *Increase of the number of undernourished people in the world. Source: FAO, IFAD, UNICEF, WFP, and WHO, "The State of Food Security and Nutrition in the World. Transforming Food Systems for Affordable Healthy", Rome, FAO (2020), p. 4.*

between 2015 and 2019. As for the estimate of malnutrition for China, the data show significantly fewer people undernourished than in 2000.

Beyond hunger, as we said, an increasing number of people do not have a suitable diet for quantity and quality and this situation could even get worse if correct initiatives are not implemented to act immediately and with courage.

However, it should be noted that globally, between 2000 and 2019, the prevalence of child stunting decreased by one-third. Nonetheless, from what has been highlighted with the data presented above, it appears that the world is not on track for achieve global nutritional goals, including those related to stunting and wasting, within the next decade.

After a decade of stable decline, the number of world people suffering from hunger has slowly increased for some years, calling attention to the huge challenge of ending hunger by 2030. The evidence available confirms that more than 800 million people in the world did not have enough to eat in 2018, which is the third year of increase in a row.[e]

Hunger is on the rise in almost all subregions of Africa, where the incidence of undernourishment has reached an intensity of 22.8% in sub-Saharan Africa, and to a lesser extent in Latin America. In Asia, although great progress in the last 5 years, Southern Asia is still the sub-region where the PoU is highest, about 15%, followed by Western Asia, at over 12%, where the situation is worsening. Looking across regions, the undernourished population is distributed unequally, with the majority living in Asia (more than 500 million). The number has been increasing progressively in Africa where it reached approximately 260 million people in 2018, with more than 90% living in sub-Saharan Africa (Fig. 7.2).

A broader investigation (FAO, IFAD, UNICEF, WFP and WHO, Rome 2019) shows that food insecurity at moderate levels involves over 17% of the world population, 1.3 billion people, without regular access to nutrients or sufficient food, but with an increased risk of various forms of malnutrition and poor health.

Furthermore, it should be noted that even if the number of stunted children declined by 10% over the past six years, this rate is well below the 50% target to be achieved by 2030. While the prevalence of stunting is declining in nearly all regions, the extent of progress varies greatly. Africa has made the least progress in reducing stunting prevalence since 2012. In 2018, Africa and Asia together accounted for more than 9 out of 10 of all

[e] See, http://www.fao.org/news/story/en/item/1200484/icode/.

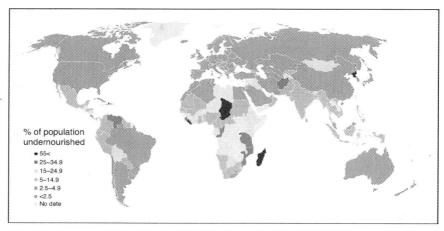

Fig. 7.2 *Percentage of population suffering from undernourishment according to United Nations Statistics (2020). Source*: https://commons.wikimedia.org/wiki/File:Percentage_population_undernourished_world_map.PNG.

stunted children globally, corresponding to 39.5% and 54.9% of the global total, respectively. The food security and nutritional status of the most vulnerable population groups is likely to deteriorate further due to the health and socio-economic impacts of the COVID-19 pandemic.

Urgent action is needed over the next decade to achieve other important global nutritional goals. Only 40% of babies under 6 months are exclusively breastfed, which is a long way off from the 2030 target of 70%. In 2018, 7.3% of the children were wasted, and this must be reduced by more than half to achieve the target of less than 3% by 2030. Anemia currently affects 33% of women of reproductive age, more than double the 2030 target of 15%. Some data relating to the weight of newborns indicate that seven out of ten live births, over 20 million children globally, they still suffer from low birth weight. Therefore, it will be difficult to achieve the goal by 2030, with a higher risk of dying in the first month of life, and those who survive are more likely to suffer from stunted growth and face an increased risk of adult-onset chronic conditions.

Further than the enormous human costs of malnutrition, the economic costs are surprising: it is expected that undernutrition will reduce Gross Domestic Product by up to 11% in Africa and Asia.

These arguments make it clear that malnutrition in all its forms is not the domain of any one sector alone. Health, education, agriculture, business community, social protection, planning, and economic policy sectors as well as legislators, institutional leaders, international organizations, researches, and academics all together have a role to play in such an important challenge.

7.3 A system thinking view to approach ethical issues in achieving SDGs

As is well known, the SDGs present an ambitious agenda, as they seek to eliminate poverty rather than reduce it, and require very demanding goals including those on health, education, gender, and equality. Compared to the MDGs, these new objectives are considered universal, since they concern all countries and all inhabitants of the world without any distinction between developed, emerging, and developing countries. However, in order that the challenges imposed by these "structural and global" ethical issues can be faced, it is proper to analyse them through a broader perspective, which includes three different dimensions: institutional, organizational, and individual, as shown in the first diagram on the left of Fig. 7.3.

The first field of analysis is focused on institutions (political, economic, social, health, etc.) aimed at preparing and implementing those mechanisms capable of preventing, mitigating or resolving economic, social, and environmental imbalances (Testa, 2007). This first dimension highlights the necessary and basic contribution of both guidelines and constraints, which at a transnational level must be clearly issued, promoted, and enforced.

The second level of investigation, on the other hand, focuses on the characteristics of the economic organizations, characterized by specific structures and diversified self-regulation mechanisms. The paradigmatic change to which increasing attention is often addressed today in relation to corporate governance is recognizable in the progressive and definitive move away from short-term logic and pure economic convenience.

The third area of search analyses the distinctive elements of the political and economic agents. They have enormous decision-making responsibilities with a role of making the principles toward a renewed sustainable development widespread and effective and, more generally, by the peculiarities of all the participants in the civil society, which with their choices are able to contribute to the path of the various institutions.

If the outlined approach in the first diagram of Fig. 7.3, presently described, appears extremely useful in order to analyse the ethical issues on which the SDGs are rooted, the second scheme of Fig. 7.3 summarizes, through the logic of the Triple Helix, the existing dynamic interaction

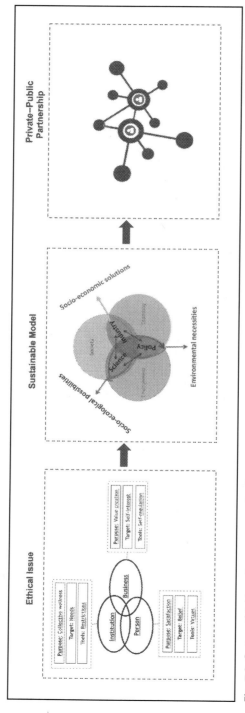

Fig. 7.3 *System thinking view to approach ethical issues.* Source: Adapted from Testa (2007) and Saviano et al. (2019).

between three actors: policy, science, and industry, as key players to achieve such crucial goals.

This approach initially originated in the model suggested in 1998 (Leydesdorff and Etzkowitz, 1998) and in 2003 (Leydesdorff and Etzkowitz, 2003) by scholars engaged in the analysis of the structural relationships existing between institutional bodies, such as universities, industry, and government, as actors having a crucial role in the effectiveness of innovation processes. Subsequent developments of this model have involved further emerging areas of research related to sustainability issues. Indeed, Saviano et al. (2019) pointed out that by adopting the perspective of sustainability, governments (policy) must take charge of the limited carrying capacity of our planet (environmental necessities), adopting measures aimed at reconciling the needs of socio-economic activities with the constraints imposed by the protection of the natural environment; science (universities/ academia) based on environmental necessities must identify the actions to be implemented in the light of scientific progress and knowledge (socio-ecological possibilities), and finally, industry must develop suitable operational answers (socio-economic solutions).

These premises reinforce the demand that arises loudly from various areas relating to the now urgent need to configure new, more integrated, and responsible business models (Barile and Saviano, 2013). The answer seems to come from public–private partnerships (PPPs), as shown in Fig. 7.3. Even if in the field of nutrition, there is no single definition of a PPP, World Health Organization (WHO) defines PPPs as "a collaboration between public-and private-sector actors within diverse arrangements that vary according to participants, legal status, governance, management, policy setting, contributions, and operational roles to achieve specific outcomes" (Fanzo et al., 2021).

In summary, in order to thoroughly analyse these ethical issues, a joint study of the various areas of observation should not be ignored and the Triple Helix model highlights the "hybridization" of the role of the various actors, which in the case study analysed was concretized in an extremely effective partnership. Moving from theory to practice, the production of the RUTFs saw the participation of university and research institutes (committed to developing innovative scientific evidence), the political world (in this case represented by United Nations agencies, able to trace an international strategic direction), and businesses (which pursuing civic purposes, solidarity, and social utility have generated a virtuous process of value cocreation).

7.4 A tool from nutraceuticals to face the Zero Hunger challenge: An overview on ready to use food (RUF)

Nutrition is a key element of healthier populations and all forms of malnutrition are risk factors with serious impact not only on premature mortality but also on human capital across the life-course. The SDGs and the United Nations Decade of Action on Nutrition (2016–2025)[f] are bringing a renewed strength for this issue, with the participation and commitment of the World Health Organization (WHO), in providing evidence-informed guidance on nutrition and healthy diets. WHO and various other institutional partners are strongly committed to actions aimed at ensuring universal access to healthy and sustainable food diets. WHO takes priority actions to improve nutrition, develop evidence-informed guidance based on sound scientific and ethical frameworks, support the adoption of guidelines and the implementation of effective actions, and monitor and evaluate the implementation of policies and programs and nutritional outcomes.[g] In 2013, the WHO released a guide entitled "Essential Nutrition Actions: improving maternal, newborn, infant and young child health and nutrition" (World Health Organization, 2013; World Health Organization, 2019) which also draws on the findings of systematic reviews such as those of the Lancet Series on Maternal and Child Undernutrition[h] to highlight the proven actions that need to be taken to scale within the health sector. Hunger is a profound obstacle to the advancement of individuals and societies, since, without proper intervention, undernutrition and death and disease it causes are repeated throughout the human life cycle (Fig. 7.4).

Over the years, the solution to the enormous problem of hunger and malnutrition in the countries at greatest risk has been identified in "ready-to-use foods" (RUFs) which are products ready to eat without

---

[f]Resolution adopted by the General Assembly on 1 April 2016: United Nations Decade of Action on Nutrition (2016–2025). In: United Nations General Assembly 70th session, 2015–2016. New York, New York: United Nations; 2016 (A/RES/70/259; http://www. un.org/en/ga/search/view_doc.asp?symbol=A/RES/70/259). The United Nations Decade of Action on Nutrition 2016–2025 focuses on action to reduce hunger and malnutrition and has recommitted Member States of WHO to achieve the WHO global nutrition targets.

[g]See, https://www.who.int/nutrition/topics/guideline-development/en/.

[h]The landmark *Lancet Series on Maternal and Child Undernutrition* published in 2008 and updated in 2013 estimated that effective, targeted nutrition interventions to address maternal and child undernutrition exist, and if implemented at scale during the 1000-day-long window of opportunity, could reduce nutrition-related mortality and disease burden by 25% (Black et al., 2013 ; Bhutta et al., 2013).

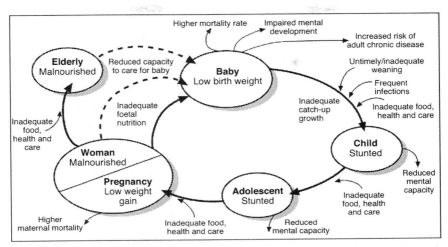

Fig. 7.4 *Effects of malnutrition throughout the life cycle. Source:* Global nutrition challenges: a life-cycle approach in Food and Nutrition Bulletin (2000).

reconstitution or preparation. As the name implies, RUF does not need to be prepared in any way prior to consumption, making it practical for use where there is contaminated water or cooking fuel and facilities are limiting constraints. Different types of products, with a variety of compositions and different applications, belong to the RUFs. Among the RUFs, the availability of ready-to-use "therapeutic" foods (RUTFs) has made it possible to achieve remarkable successes in-home therapies. They are usually made of powdered ingredients embedded in a lipid-rich paste, resulting in an energy-dense food that resists microbial contamination (Godswill et al. 2020; Manary et al., 2004; Collins and Sadler, 2003; Briend, 2002). These products have a high nutrient density, about 23 kJ/g (5.5 kcal/g), and a low propensity for bacterial growth even without refrigeration and, in addition, they need no cooking or other preparation and can be fed directly from their packaging with no need for training (Manary, 2005; Schoones et al., 2019).

This allows locally produced RUTFs to be safely stored at ambient tropical conditions for 3–4 months. A severely malnourished child can consume just a few spoonfuls of RUTF 5–7 times a day, and achieve sufficient nutrient intake for complete recovery and, consumed with water, no other foods are necessary for the rehabilitation (Manary, 2005). Indeed in 2007 WHO, in collaboration with the United Nations Children's Fund (UNICEF), the World Food Programme (WFP), and the United Nations System Standing Committee on Nutrition (UNSSC) released a Joint Statement on community-based management of severe acute malnutrition (SAM) which recommends that children with uncomplicated SAM be treated with RUTF. The organizations involved in RUTFs production should adhere to the standards set by FAO and WHO in the Codex Alimentarius (Codex Alimentarius Commission, 2017; Codex Alimentarius Commission, 2020) and related updates. Generally, RUTFs are spreadable preparations that require simple production technologies, transferable to countries with not very advanced industrial infrastructures. However, there are other technologies that could eventually be transferred to countries with more advanced industrial capabilities. Comparison of standard RUTF versus an alternative dietary approach (e.g., flour porridge or locally available foods) in severely malnourished children aged 6 months to 5 years and key health outcomes show recovery from severe malnutrition, deterioration or relapse, death, and the rate of weight gain (Schoonees et al., 2019). Among RUFs, while the RUTFs are generally used in the treatment of SAM, the ready-to-use "supplemental" foods (RUSFs) are being tested for more widespread use either in the treatment of moderate acute malnutrition (MAM) or for replacing other foods used in food aid. The "lipid-based nutritional supplements" are a type of RUSF with reduced bulk, currently investigated as an alternative that could minimize the risk of displacing breastmilk. In terms of value, the global RUTF and RUSF market is estimated at around 430 Mn US dollars in 2017, and expected to reach around 830 Mn US dollars by 2025 (news provided by Transparency Market Research, 2017).

7.5 Ready to use therapeutic food (RTUTF): Opportunities and constraints

7.5.1 Background

Malnourished children usually have a high risk of illness and death. Treat severely malnourished children in hospitals is not always feasible especially in rural contexts, so home treatment may prove to be a better approach, through the use of RUTFs. The introduction of RUTFs in the management of SAM has allowed health authorities to expand effective treatment beyond hospitals, that is, in out-patient units or at home, thus significantly reducing cost and the burden on in-patient health care facilities, and allowing an amplified coverage. Unfortunately, this approach based on a more sustainable model is far from universal and in many cases, sometimes the worst ones, are not yet achieved by related programs. They are usually produced on the basis of a "standard" energy-rich composition defined by the World Health Organization (WHO)[i] with precise amounts of micronutrients, providing energy equivalent to WHO requirement (i.e., 520–550 kcal/100 g) (Wagh and Deore, 2015). The RUTFs have a nutritional composition similar to the F-100 (100 kcal per 100 ml), a therapeutic milk product used in the hospital to treat SAM. Generally, their composition requires that at least half of the proteins contained in RUTFs should come from milk products (World Health Organization, World Food Programme, United Nations System Standing Committee on Nutrition, The United Nations Children's Fund, 2007). Typically, the ingredients for standard RUTF include milk powder, sugar, peanut butter, vegetable oil, vitamins, and minerals. However, ingredients may vary enormously depending on local availability, cost, and acceptability.

The RUTFs present some problems related to the unsuitable storage and handling of raw materials and products; indeed, for instance, the peanut butter can be contaminated by aflatoxins that are carcinogenic molecules (Awad et al., 2012; Barberis et al., 2012; Santini et al., 2013).

Recently, alternative RUTF formulations with reduced milk protein, or no milk protein, have been evaluated in different researches, with the aim to reduce the production cost by replacing milk (the most expensive ingredient and more often imported) with other less expensive sources of energy, protein, and other important nutrients. A decision tree (Fig. 7.5) was developed in order to guide decision-making for evidence on acceptability, efficacy, and effectiveness of an alternative RUTF based on compliance with the Joint Statement (UNICEF, 2021). The alternative formulations of a RUTF are known under the category of "renovation" products, as they represent a step-change in the ingredients habitually used. They can be formed using the same processes and the established equipment and manufacturing of traditional RUTFs.

The most common alternative ingredients are based on some main resources, as cereals, protein sources that can be of plant (beans, legumes, etc.) or animal (milk, red or white meat, fish meat, egg, etc.) origin, energetic supplements (lipids, oil, sugar, etc.), mineral and vitamin supplements (derived from vegetal, fruits, or a mixture of both), and nutraceuticals (Collins and Henry, 2004; Santini et al., 2013; Wagh and Deore, 2015). The economic saving allows the treatment of a greater number of children with SAM, to an extent that currently is about 25%. However, the results obtained from the use of alternative RTUFs show, on the one hand, an efficacy similar to the standard ones in terms of recovery, mortality, and rate of weight gain, but on the other hand, their use is not as effective in preventing relapses (Schoonees et al., 2019). In recent years, various institutions and

---

[1]In 2007, WHO, in collaboration with the United Nations Children's Fund (UNICEF), the World Food Programme (WFP), and the United Nations System Standing Committee on Nutrition (UNSSC) released a Joint Statement on *Community-based management of severe acute malnutrition (SAM)* which recommends that children with uncomplicated SAM be treated with ready-to-use therapeutic foods (RUTFs).

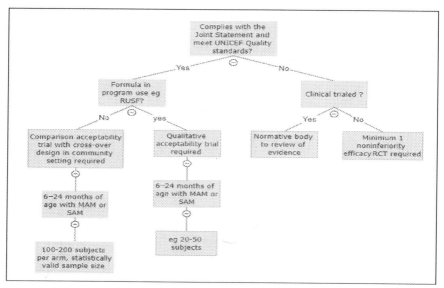

Fig. 7.5 *Decision tree for deciding which kind of evidence is needed for new RUTF formulations. Source*: https://www.unicef.org/supply/media/3316/file/RUTF-technical-expert-meeting-report-02-03092019.pdf.pdf>.

numerous researchers have been engaging to scientifically evaluate the efficacy, safety, acceptability, and cost of formulations of alternative RUTFs used in the treatment of infants and children aged 6 or older months with SAM. This is in line with the goals of the 2025 World Health Assembly and the 2030 SDGs to end preventable deaths of infants and children under 5 of age.

7.5.2 Market

The first commercially available RUTFs were produced in the late 1980s and patented in 1993 by the French firm Nutriset[j] under the commercial name Plumpy'nut, containing peanuts, milk powder, sugar, oil, and vitamin and mineral mix. The development of RUTFs and the implementation of highly effective program model of home-based therapy for the treatment of SAM, namely Community-based Management of Acute Malnutrition (CMAM), have significantly increased the effectiveness of therapeutic feeding care and enabled increased beneficiary access (WHO/WFP/United Nations System Standing Committee on Nutrition/UNICEF, 2007). The success has led to a surge in their demand especially in low–income countries characterized by greater food insecurity due to environmental factors

[j]See https://www.nutriset.fr/en/history.

Table 7.1 UNICEF supply arrangements for RUTF in 2019–2021 (2023 for RUTF biscuits).

	Supplier	Type of supply	Start	End	Product
1	Amul Dairy (Kaira), India	International	Apr-19	Apr-21	RUTF Paste
2	Compact, India	International	Apr-19	Apr-21	RUTF Paste
3	DABS Nigeria	Local	Apr-19	Apr-21	RUTF Paste
4	Diva Nutritional Products, South Africa	International	Apr-19	Apr-21	RUTF Paste
5	Edesia, USA	International	Apr-19	Apr-21	RUTF Paste
6	GC Rieber Compact, Norway	International	May-20	May-23	RUTF Biscuits
7	GC Rieber Compact, South Africa	International	Apr-19	Apr-21	RUTF Paste
8	Hexagon, India	International	Apr-20	Apr-21	RUTF Paste
9	Hilina, Ethiopia	Local	Apr-19	Apr-21	RUTF Paste
10	InnoFaso, Burkina Faso	International/Local	Apr-19	Apr-21	RUTF Paste
11	Insta Products, Kenya	International/Local	Apr-19	Apr-21	RUTF Paste
12	Ismail Industries, Pakistan	International/Local	Apr-19	Apr-21	RUTF Paste
13	Mana Nutritive Aid, USA	International	May-20	Apr-21	RUTF Paste
14	Meds for Kids, Haiti	International/Local	Apr-19	Apr-21	RUTF Paste
15	Nuflower Foods and Nutrition, India	International	May-20	Apr-21	RUTF Paste
16	Nutriset, France	International	Apr-19	Apr-21	RUTF Paste
17	NutriVita Foods, India	International	May-20	Apr-21	RUTF Paste
18	Project Peanut Butter, Malawi	Local	Apr-19	Apr-21	RUTF Paste
19	Samil Industry, Sudan	International/Local	Apr-19	Apr-21	RUTF Paste
20	Société de Transformation Alimentaire, Niger	International/Local	Apr-19	Apr-21	RUTF Paste
21	Société JB, Madagascar	International/Local	Apr-19	Apr-21	RUTF Paste
22	Soma Nutrition, India	International	Apr-20	Apr-21	RUTF Paste

Sources: UNICEF Supply Division (2021), Ready to use therapeutic food: market outlook. https://www.unicef.org/supply/media/7256/file/RUTF-Supply-Update-March-2021.pdf.

such as cyclical drought (Bazzano et al., 2017). Nutriset's patent initially did not help local production in low-income contexts where instead RUTFs were most needed, so in 2005 Nutriset developed PlumpyField Network, a worldwide network of franchisees in programmatic countries producing Plumpy'nut under license[k]. Further, in 2010 Nutriset implemented a patent use agreement for producers in selected developing countries where the company held a patent to manufacture in order to facilitate local production of peanut-based RUTF. As this additional capacity could not satisfy ever-growing demand, UNICEF advocated with food manufacturers to start production of generic RUTFs and, currently, there are more than 20 UNICEF-approved manufacturers of peanut-based RUTFs (Table 7.1), and 18 suppliers are localized in countries with high levels of malnutrition.

At present UNICEF[l] is the most important procurer: 75%–80% of the global demand for RUTFs, supplying these products to over 55 countries (Fig. 7.6).

[k]The PlumpyField network (Nutriset. The PlumpyField Network: How it works) plays a singular role bringing together independent franchised contractors operating in countries affected by malnutrition and promoting their sustainable development through the use of local agricultural resources and the deployment of agri-industrial activity. Since its inception in 2005, the network, which now has 12 members, has supported 60 million children. Its current members are: Edesia (USA), Hexagon Nutrition (India), Hilina Enriched Foods (Ethiopia), InnoFaso (Burkina Faso), Meds and Food for Kids (Haiti), Nutriguinée (Guinea), Nutri-K/Dansa (Nigeria), Nutriset (France), Nutrivita Foods (India), Samil (Sudan), Food Processing Society (Niger), Tanjaka Food (Madagascar). See http://www.plumpyfield.com/about/how-it-works. See http://www.plumpyfield.com/about/how-it-works.

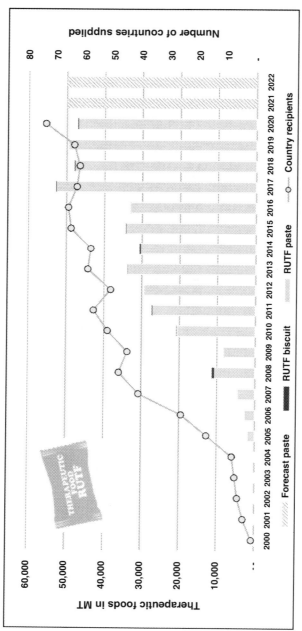

Fig. 7.6 *UNICEF RUTF Procurement, Forecast, and Number of Countries Supplied 2000–2022. Source:* UNICEF Supply Division (2021), Ready to Use Therapeutic Food: Market Outlook. https://www.unicef.org/supply/media/7256/file/RUTF-Supply-Update-March-2021.pdf.

The residual global volumes are procured directly by governments, other UN agencies (UNHCR, WHO), and other main international organizations. UNICEF exceeded the target of sourcing at least 50% of RUTF from suppliers located in program countries at the end of 2016 reaching 56% and increasing this level to over 70% in 2020 (Fig. 7.7).

In 2020, the total volume of RUTFs and other supplementary lipid-based nutrition products procured reached around 140,000 Mt. Unfortunately, it is estimated that the economic consequences of the Covid 19 pandemic, in addition to problems in routine health and nutrition services, are leading to increased levels of malnutrition.[m] In such a scenario, both UNICEF and WFP will work with national governments and nutrition agencies to support the design and scale-up of simplified and specific approaches for early recognition and treatment of child wasting.

In February 2018, UNICEF approved a procedure on "sustainable procurement", an approach incorporating the three sustainability pillars of social, economic, and environmental impact concerns. This approach goes beyond the more common "green" procurement, ensuring that all products and services procured sustain local economy and social development with the least environment impact and at the best value for money (UNICEF, Supply Division 2021). To support the many initiatives already planned and implemented by RUTF manufacturers, UNICEF will monitor progress on sustainability with due consideration for the health of the market and the finished product's affordability.

The main challenge still to be faced is to strongly promote the RUTFs production locally, in such a way to bring the product closer to the needs of beneficiary and thereby facilitate the transfer of CMAM program management from NGO/UN agencies to National Governments.

---

[l] UNICEF places two types of orders for RUTF: nonemergency and emergency. Nonemergency orders are planned in advance, while the demands of RUTF in emergencies make forecasts very challenging and often inaccurate. In 2013, the Nutrition Dashboard (NutriDash) was created to address these challenges effectively. Furthermore, emergency orders are often shipped via air freight, an expensive approach that imposes trade-offs between decreasing lead time and minimizing costs. la

[m] See, https://data.unicef.org/resources/impacts-of-covid-19-on-childhood-malnutrition-and-nutrition-related-mortality/ and https://www.unicef.org/press-releases/nutrition-crisis-looms-more-39-billion-school-meals-missed-start-pandemic-unicef-and.

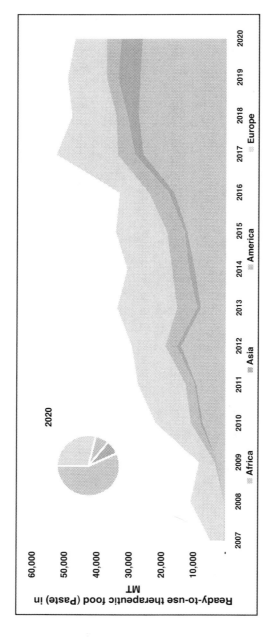

Fig. 7.7 *UNICEF RUTF (Paste) Procurement by Production Region of Origin 2007–2020. Source:* UNICEF Supply Division (2021), Ready to Use Therapeutic Food: Market Outlook. https://www.unicef.org/supply/media/7256/file/RUTF-Supply-Update-March-2021.pdf.

Locally produced RUTFs not require shipment via long and consequently complex supply chains and procurement from local manufactures reduce lead times and shipping costs, contributing to improve sustainability by reducing transportation carbon footprint and providing economic development opportunities. Unfortunately, such an approach is hindered by reliance on imported products with lower costs, as local manufacturers have higher production costs as they have to pay taxes on imports of raw material used, high-interest rates, and face costs for the long cycle of cash conversion, as well as difficulties related to accessing laboratories for the necessary tests quality (Segré et al., 2016). Although the weighted average price (WAP) of RUTFs from local suppliers, both franchisees and independent, decreased from USD 60.00 per carton[n] in 2009 to fall below USD 49.00 in 2017, with a decrease of 20% over eight years (UNICEF Supply Division, 2019), and 45.64 in 2020 (UNICEF Supply Division 2021), currently it is 12%–14% higher than that from international suppliers (Fig. 7.8).

Nevertheless, as regard domestic production, the market has witnessed a rapid upsurge since the past decade, and a growing trend is expected also due to the UNICEF initiatives for the research and development of alternative raw materials produced locally and efforts are underway to narrow the cost gap further. According to the report "Ready-to-use Therapeutic Food Market: Global Industry Analysis and Forecast, 2018–2026"[o] RUTF market is estimated to growth at a CAGR of around 10.3% throughout the outlook period of 2021–2026. The regional analysis highlights constant dominance of the European market, primarily because the European companies have been the key providers of RUTFs to leading organizations, such as UNICEF[p]. Among the leading players in the global RUTF market there are Compact AS Diva Nutritional Products (South Africa), Edesia USA, Hilina (Ethopia), InnoFaso (Burkina Faso), Insta Products (Kenya), Mana Nutritive Aid Products (USA), Nutriset SAS (France), NutriVita Foods (India), Power Foods Tanzania, Samil Industrial (Sudan), Tabatchnik Fine Food (USA).

---

[n]One carton contains 150 sachets of 92g., 72 cartons make up 1 Mt.

[o]See https://www.marketdataforecast.com/market-reports/ready-to-use-therapeutic-food-market.

[p]See https://soccernurds.com/uncategorized/939146/ready-to-use-therapeutic-food-market-to-witness-significant-rise-in-revenue-during-the-forecast-period-2024/.

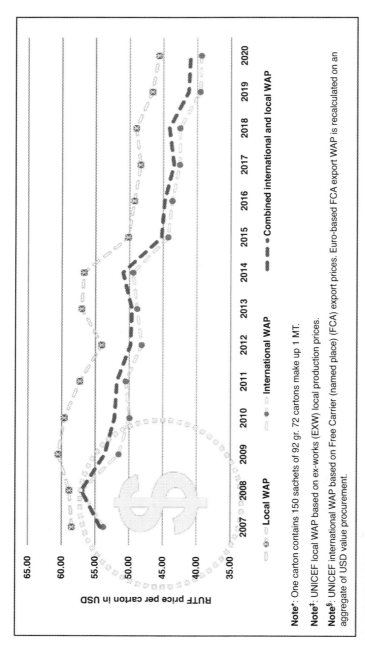

Note*: One carton contains 150 sachets of 92 gr. 72 cartons make up 1 MT.

Note‡: UNICEF local WAP based on ex-works (EXW) local production prices.

Note§: UNICEF international WAP based on Free Carrier (named place) (FCA) export prices. Euro-based FCA export WAP is recalculated on an aggregate of USD value procurement.

Fig. 7.8 *UNICEF WAP for International and Local RUTF Paste Procurement 2007–2020. Source:* UNICEF Supply Division (2021), Ready to Use Therapeutic Food: Market Outlook. https://www.unicef.org/supply/media/7256/file/RUTF-Supply-Update-March-2021.pdf.

7.6 Conclusions

Shared value derives from different ways of involvement, such as philanthropic and corporate social responsibility, market definition, product innovation, and strategic procurement. To address Zero Poverty and Hunger targets by 2030 Agenda for Sustainable Development, the creation of shared values cannot be separated from the involvement of multiple forces, establishing a framework for identifying opportunities to improve socioeconomic and environmental outcomes and related performance (Polese et al., 2015; Lush et al., 2017). Value cocreation, through the distribution of RUTFs, means optimizing the results for a good and regular growth of children and for the well-being of their families. Furthermore, this approach provides business organizations with an opportunity to enter new markets, supporting economies, and promoting sustainability. The SDGs offer an excellent framework for global growth and prosperity and the commitment to realize shared values can offer benefits and growth opportunities especially in terms of social impact. It is, therefore, all the more important to act jointly on the basis of shared vision, because valid responses to such crucial challenges require the strong commitment of many actors. They range from economic organizations through the emblematic tools of corporate social responsibility to international organizations through effective philanthropic initiatives, from researchers to develop and encourage process and product innovations suitable for different contexts identifying problems and supporting more local production to governmental institutions and humanitarian organizations to outline a clear and transparent framework in order to face logistic, legal and financial challenges for the successful operation of these new markets. Africa is one of those regions that have enormous margins for development and that can make a decisive contribution to the realization of a new paradigm of sustainable development. In addition, many of the problems highlighted above are closely related to each other and in a cause-effect relationship. With reference to the financial aspect, access to useful and safe financial services has the potential to empower women especially and thus improve the food security of their family members (Testa and Pellicano, 2018). The pervasiveness of financial services designed to alleviate poverty can improve the problem of undernutrition, as the development of their multiple applications can only help to promote economic and social development and for this reason, it is key to achieving SDG2 targets. In fact, financial inclusion, facilitating access to health treatments useful for food security, constitutes a notable support for the reduction of malnutrition and in particular of childhood undernutrition (World Health Organization, 2018).

Hence, adopting a more concrete perspective, the PPPs represent a good and operative synthesis of the above. The implementation of PPPs in order to contribute to the solution of the serious problem of undernutrition seems to have broad prospects of benefits, as it can stimulate private investment and supplementary resources to promote development and support local food and agricultural systems, in order to increase products, expand capacity and lower pricing for life-saving supplies. Furthermore, alongside the commitment of governments and institutions and the advancement of knowledge by universities and research centres, the participation of the private sector could be useful in driving innovative processes aimed at improving the affordability and availability of the procurement cycle rooted in the territory with the chance to optimize the functioning of the short supply chain for RUTFs, the assessment of leakage problems and quality issues.

References

Awad, W.A., Ghareeb, K., Bohm, J., 2012. Occurrence, health risks and methods of analysis for aflatoxins and ochratoxin A. J. Veterinary Animal Sci. 2, 1–10.

Barberis, C.L., Dalcero, A.M., Magnoli, C.E., 2012. Evaluation of aflatoxin B1 and ochratoxin A in interacting mixed cultures of Aspergillus sections Flavi and Nigri on peanut grains. Mycotoxin Res. http://doi.org/10.1007/s12550-012-0126-y.

Barile, S., Saviano, M., 2013. An introduction to a value co-creation model, viability, syntropy and resonance in dyadic interaction. Syntropy 2 (2), 69–89.

Bazzano, A.N., Potts, K.S., Bazzano, L.A., Mason, J.B., April 2017. The life course implications of ready to use therapeutic food for children in low-income countries. Int. J. Environ. Res. Public Health 14, 403. doi:10.3390/ijerph14040403 www.mdpi.com/journal/ijerph.

Bhutta, Z.A., Das, J.K., Rizvi, A., Gaffey, M.F., Walker, N., Horton, S., Webb, P., Lartey, A., Black, R.E., 2013. Evidence-based interventions for improvement of maternal and child nutrition: what can be done and at what cost? Lancet North Am. Ed. 382 (9890), 452–477. DOI. http://doi.org/10.1016/S0140-6736(13)60996-4.

Black, R.E., Victora, C.G., Walker, S.P., Bhutta, Z.A., Christian, P., de Onis, M., Ezzati, M., Ghrantam-McGregor, S., Katz, J., Martorell, R., Uauy, R., 2013. Maternal and child undernutrition and overweight in low-income and middle-income countries. The Lancet 382 (9890), 427–451. https://doi.org/10.1016/S0140-6736(13)60937-X.

Briend, A., 2002. Possible use of spreads as a FOODlet for improving the diets of infants and young children. Food Nutr Bull 23 (3), 239–243.

Codex Alimentarius Commission (2017), Joint FAO/WHO Food standards programme codex committee on nutrition and foods for special dietary uses, CX/NFSDU 17/39/7-Add.1, Berlin 2017.

Codex Alimentarius Commission (2020), Joint FAO/WHO Food standards programme codex alimentarius commission, REP20/NFSDU, Rome

Collins, S. and Henry, J., 2004. "Alternative RUTF Formulations (Special Supplement 2)," Field Exchange, no. 102.

Collins, S., Sadler, K., 2003. Outpatient care for severely malnourished children in emergency relief programmes: a retrospective cohort study. Lancet North Am. Ed. 360 (9348). http://doi.org/10.1016/S0140-6736(02)11770-3.

Fanzo, J., Shawar, Y.R., Shyam, T., Das, S., Shiffman, J., 2021. Challenges to establish effective Public-Private-Partnerships to address malnutrition in all its forms. Int. J. Health Policy Manag., 1–12.

FAO, IFAD, UNICEF, WFP and WHO, 2019. The State of Food Security and Nutrition in the World 2019. Safeguarding against economic slowdowns and downturns. FAO, Rome Licence: CC BY-NC-SA 3.0 IGOISSN 2663-8061, CA5162EN/1/07.19.

FAO, IFAD, UNICEF, WFP and WHO. 2020. The State of Food Security and Nutrition in the World 2020. Transforming food systems for affordable healthy diets. Rome, FAO. https://doi.org/10.4060/ca9692en

Food and Nutrition Bulletin. Supplement December 2021. The United Nations University. https://journals.sagepub.com/doi/pdf/10.1177/15648265000213S104.

Godswill, A.C, Somtochukwu, I.V., Ikechukwu, A., 2020. Ready-to-use therapeutic foods (RUTFs) for remedying malnutrition and preventable nutritional diseases. Int. J. Adv. Academic Res. Sci., Technol. Eng. 6 (1) ISSN: 2488-98492020.

http://www.fao.org/fao-who-codexalimentarius/sh-proxy/en/?lnk=1&url=https%253A%252F%252Fworkspace.fao.org%252Fsites%252Fcodex%252FMeetings%252FCX-720-39%252Fnf39_01_rev1e.pdf

http://www.fao.org/fao-who-codexalimentarius/sh-proxy/en/?lnk=1&url=https%253A%252F%252Fworkspace.fao.org%252Fsites%252Fcodex%252FMeetings%252FCX-720-41%252FReport%252FAdoption%252FREP20_NFSDUe.pdf

Leydesdorff, L., Etzkowitz, H., 1998. The triple helix as a model for innovation studies. Sci Public Policy 25 (3), 195–203.

Leydesdorff, L., Etzkowitz, H., 2003. Can 'the public' be considered as a fourth helix in university–industry–government relations? Report on the fourth triple helix conference, 2002 Science and Public Policy, 30, 55–61.

Lusch, R.F., Vargo, S.L., Mele, C., Polese, F., "Service-dominant logic: premesse, prospettive, possibilità", Cedam, 2017

Manary, M.J., (December 2001). Technical Background Paper. Local production and provision of ready-to-use therapeutic food for the treatment of severe childhood malnutrition. https://www.who.int/nutrition/topics/backgroundpapers_Local_production.pdf.

Manary, M.J., Ndekha, M.J., Ashorn, P., et al., 2004. Home-based therapy for severe malnutrition with ready-to-use-food. Arch Dis Child 2004 89 (6), 557–561.

Nutriset. The PlumpyField Network: How It Works. http://www.nutriset.fr/en/plumpy-field/plumpyfield-how-it-works.html (December 2021).

Polese, F., Iandolo, F., Carrubbo, L., 2015. Co-creare valore compartecipando valori. Un contributo in ottica service tra fruizione e compartecipazione, Conference Proceeding XXVII Convegno annuale di Sinergie, Heritage Management e impresa: quali sinergie? 317–335.

Santini, A., Novellino, E., Armini, V., Ritieni, A., 2013. State of the art of ready-to-use therapeutic food: a tool for nutraceuticals addition to foodstuff. Food Chem. 140 (4), 843–849.

Saviano, M., Barile, S., Farioli, F., Orecchini, F., 2019. Strengthening the science–policy–industry interface for progressing toward sustainability: a systems thinking view. Sustainability Sci. 14, 1549–1564. https://doi.org/10.1007/s11625-019-00668-x.

Schoonees, A., Lombard, M.J., Musekiwa, A., Nel, E., Volmink, J., 2019. Ready-to-use therapeutic food (RUTF) for home-based nutritional rehabilitation of severe acute malnutrition in children from six months to five years of age. *Cochrane Database of Systematic Reviews* 2019. Published by John Wiley&Sons, Ltd. Art. No.: CD009000. http://doi.org/10.1002/14651858.CD009000.pub3 The Cochrane Collaboration.

Segrè, J., Liu, G., Komrska, J., 2016. Local versus offshore production of ready-to-use therapeutic foods and small quantity lipid-based nutrient supplements. Matern Child Nutr. http://doi.org/10.1111/mcn.12376.

Testa, M., 2007. La Responsabilità Sociale d'Impresa. Aspetti strategici, modelli di analisi e strumenti operativi. Giappichelli, Torino ISBN 978-88-348-7737-1.

Testa, M., Pellicano, M., 2018. *Mobile Transactions: a powerful channel to drive financial inclusion.* Evidence from Kenya: M-PESA Model. In: Tesar, G., Anderson, S.W., Traore, H., Graff, J. (Eds.), Marketing management in Africa. Routledge, London.

Transparency Market Research, https://www.transparencymarketresearch.com/rutf-rusf-market.html (December 2021).

UNICEF Supply Division, 2019, Ready to use therapeutic food: market outlook. https://www.unicef.org/supply/media/7251/file/RUTF-Supply-Update-December-2021.pdf

UNICEF Supply Division, 2021, Ready to use therapeutic food: market outlook. https://www.unicef.org/supply/media/7256/file/RUTF-Supply-Update-December-2021.pdf.

Wagh, V.D., Deore, B.R., 2015. Ready to use Therapeutic Food (RTUTF): an overview. Adv. Life Sci. Health 2 (1).

WHO/WFP/United Nations System Standing Committee on Nutrition/UNICEF, 2007, Community-Based Management of Severe Acute Malnutrition, A Joint Statement by the World Health Organization, the World Food Programme, the United Nations System Standing Committee on Nutrition and the United Nations Children's Fund. ISBN: 978-92-806-4147-9

World Health Organization, 2019. Essential nutrition actions: mainstreaming nutrition through the life-course. World Health Organization, Geneva. Licence: CC BY-NC-SA 3.0 IGO. ISBN 978-92-4-151585-6.

World Health Organization; 2018. Licence: CC BY-NC-SA 3.0 IGO. ISBN 978-92-4-151364-7

World Health Organization, 2013. Essential Nutrition Actions: Improving Maternal, Newborn, Infant and Young Child Health and Nutrition. Geneva ISBN 978 92 4 150555 0 (NLM classification: WD 100).

CHAPTER 8

Typical plant-based food from a nutraceutical perspective: The case of the Marche region

Gianni Sagratini[a], Cristina Santini[b], Giovani Caprioli[a], Sauro Vittori[a], Filippo Maggi[a], Astride Franks Kamgang Nzekoue[a], Riccardo Petrelli[a]
[a]School of Pharmacy, Universiy of Camerino, Camerino, Italy
[b]University San Raffaele Rome, Italy

8.1 Nutraceutical food plants and strategy

Nutraceuticals grew in popularity even because of their efficacy in terms of health benefits. Research that explores the role of nutraceuticals for health purposes is growing.

Nasri et al. (2014) highlight the relevance that nutraceuticals might have as an alternative for pharmaceuticals.

The growing interest and demand for superfoods and nutraceuticals have created a new market space for local producers. In some countries, the availability of locally grown plants that bring health benefits has created the base for competitive territorial advantage.

Furthermore, there is a strong linkage between local culture, natural resources, and employment for healthy purposes. The knowledge of natural resources and the health benefits of plants characterises many cultures and local populations.

Background research outlines the relevance of knowledge of nutraceutical dishes for rural areas and populations. This issue particularly emerges from Sujarwo et al. (2014), who focus on the indigenous Balinese population and outline how globalisation could threaten folk knowledge of natural resources.

Thus, the availability of specific types of plants that fit with some diets can become leverage for local development.

Following the emerging insights from background research, we can say that recovering the nutraceutical aspects of local plants would improve resistance to cultural erosion due to globalisation. In particular, the ongoing globalisation process could threaten the cultural heritage represented by the diffused knowledge of local plants, as we can see in the work by Sujarwo et al. (2014).

Given the growing market demand, we can say that local plants with healthy and nutraceutical properties can leverage the development of rural communities. Furthermore, nutraceutical features of plants can be strategically employed for rejuvenating mature products.

8.2 Nutraceuticals plants in the Marche region

The Marche region is in the central part of Italy. The regional economy finds food, handcrafts, wine one of its pillars. The region sees many small and medium enterprises organised in industrial clusters. The Marche region has 16 gastronomic products registered as the protected denomination of origin (PDO), protected geographical indication (PGI), or traditional specialties guaranteed (TSG), 21 such as wines, and 152 other products that are very well known locally (Aleffi and Cavicchi, 2021). Some of these products are of vegetable origin as Mela Rosa dei Monti Sibillini (an ancient variety of apple), Anice verde di Castignano (a local ecotype of aniseed), Cicerchia di Serra dè Conti (a kind of pulse), Lenticchia di Castelluccio di Norcia (a kind of lentil) that is produced in a territory between Marche and Umbria regions. Typical food should be considered from a nutritional point of view, its history, and its traditional characteristics and as a source of bioactive substances useful for human health to prevent or reduce the incidence of diseases. The word "nutraceutical" was firstly introduced by the pharmacologist Stephen de Felice in 1990, and it is not regulated yet. It describes a molecule, a concentrated mix of natural substances or food that exhibits a beneficial effect on human health. Animal and vegetable foods could be considered "nutraceuticals" when they or their by-products contain substances capable of exerting relevant effects on the physiology of organisms once consumed through a regular diet.

Wandjou et al. (2020) evaluated the nutraceutical potential of the Mela Rosa dei Monti Sibillini (MR), an ancient apple variety of the Sibillini Mountains (Marche Region), by determining 21 phytochemicals and studying the antioxidant activity of a polyphenolic rich extract.

Iannarelli et al. (2017) investigated the nutraceutical potential of Castignano aniseed (Pimpinella anisum) for its possible valorisation in the local economy. Morresi et al. (2018) characterised the nutritional composition of 11 apple varieties (Malus Domestica), including nine varieties from the Regional Repertory of Biodiversity of the Marche region. They studied the antioxidant activity of apple extracts on glycoloxidative stress. Cappelletti et al. (2013) identified and characterised three artichoke landraces (Montelupone A, Precoce di Jesi, Violetto di Pesaro) typically cultivated in different districts of the Marche area, by determining the morphological characteristics, the chemical composition, the antioxidant capacity, and the polyphenolic content, in order to evaluate their potential as nutraceuticals or functional foods. Lucchetti et al. (2019) published a survey in which the ethnobotanical, medicinal, and food uses of 195 species (wild and cultivated) coming from the Marche region have been investigated. Vila Donat et al. (2014) reported the study and determination of soyasaponins I and beta g in 30 different samples of lentils coming from Marche and Umbria regions; those molecules have an interesting profile, with an evident hypocholesterolemic effect. Iannarelli et al. (2017) studied the aniseed (Pimpinella anisum) from Castignano (Marche), extensively cultivated in central Italy in the XIX century and abandoned after the global market favoured other products. In particular, the authors have produced and chemically characterised the essential oils from aniseed, and they have investigated the phenolic composition.

8.3 The strategic process of mature product rejuvenation

Product life cycle (PLC) is characterised by phases, from its introduction to its maturity.

Background literature has widely explored the concept of PLC. Some works have outlined the relationships between profitability, competitiveness, strategy, and PLC.

Anderson and Zeithaml (1984) work represents a milestone in the field. Maturity, in general, is not associated with high-performing strategies. When a product reaches the maturity stage, producing companies focus on efficiency improvement to reduce costs associated with production or distribution. Mature products have a long presence on the market, and their growth rate is steady or lower than the one registered at the initial stages.

In the case of products distinguished by high contents of technology, the stage of maturity happens earlier when compared to low-tech products.

Background research describes the dynamics of high-tech products where research and development facilitate introducing new products in the market (see among the others Cutler and Ozawa, 2007). The above-described situation contributes to shortening the length of PLC.

For many companies, mature products represent a source of income, and when companies find a way to differentiate their products from competitors, this represents a way to achieve profitability (Andrews and Smith, 1996).

The above-described scenario fits particularly well with the competitive environment of the agrifood industry, and more specifically, with food-producing companies.

In general, researchers describe the food processing industry as a mature, slow-growing industry with a low level of R&D (Costa and Jongen, 2006; Sarkar and Costa, 2008). Therefore, market trends and emerging consumers' demands stimulate companies to innovate.

In this scenario, nutraceuticals emerge and play a crucial role in reshaping the food industry's competitive dynamics.

In particular, companies that operate in the food industry or other industries, such as the pharmaceutical, can develop nutraceutical products. There is a convergence occurring in the industry between food and pharmaceuticals (Bröring et al., 2006), which stimulates the development of new products that answer emerging consumers' needs (see among the others Gul et al., 2016; Naylor et al., 2009).

In some cases, the association between food and health benefits can differentiate a product from competitors. Thus, the continuous search for food whose consumption is associated with health benefits has opened new market possibilities for food producers.

The work by Bonanno (2013) describes how yoghurt producers have differentiated their product portfolio with the introduction of functional yoghurt; this represents a case of differentiation pursued by exploring the possibilities offered by nutraceutical components when associated with yoghurt, a traditional and widely diffused (or mature) food product.

It emerges how nutraceutical aspects of food can help revitalise mature products or local productions. In this paragraph, we will explore two issues that can have a crucial role in revitalising mature products: the first is the relationship between consumer's health concerns and local product consumption; the second is the linkage between traditional food culture and the diffused knowledge about beneficial properties of local foods.

8.3.1 Consumers, health, and local products

Consumers show a growing interest in food with some recognised healthy properties. The emerging trends—such as the aging of the population, the accessibility of information about medical evidence, the role of media (Goldberg, 2012)—have nurtured consumers' interest in functional properties in food. Therefore, in some countries, the availability of nutraceutical foods associated with healthy food consumption habits has represented an opportunity for local producers to differentiate their products. One example is the one proposed in Rivera et al. (2005): the authors underline the positive role that Mediterranean food plants have played in local development in the Castilla regions in southern Spain. The Mediterranean Diet Paradigm, which is fully coherent with the emerging need for healthy food consumption, has stimulated interest in local products that contain virtuous properties. The regions of La Mancha and Lower Segura Valley, as Rivera et al. (2005) suggest, are characterised by the availability of plants that are part of the local (Mediterranean) diet and belong to traditional cuisine.

Alarcòn et al. (2015) underline the strong linkage between cultural issues and the massive employment of food plants by local heritage, and Heinrich et al. (2005) have studied the implementation of nutraceutical plants in typical food recipes and the diffusion of related knowledge among local populations in the Mediterranean area.

Recent studies confirm that marketing can successfully employ the concepts of "Mediterranean food" and "Mediterranean Diet" in food products promotion (Jiménez-Morales and Blasco, 2021). Therefore, when marketing typical food products, companies can focus on nutraceutical food properties and the role of products in local culture and tradition.

Some food products are essential resources for healthy food consumption habits: the Mediterranean diet is an example.

The topic of the relationship between health and food finds an endless debate in the academic literature, and it has been examined from different points of view and approaches.

In this chapter, we want to outline how the healthy features of a specific food product can be employed when designing a marketing strategy. Background research suggests that consumers generally consider Health Claims when they buy food. However, they must understand the meaning of the message promoted by the health claim (see among the others the work by Van Buul and Brouns, 2015).

The paper published by Basu et al. (2007) outlines how companies employ nutraceutical properties of selected local food products to develop niche market strategies and improve local producers' competitiveness.

8.3.2 Local food properties and traditional food knowledge

Another exciting aspect is the relationship between traditions, food culture, and local/typical dishes that employ food with nutraceutical properties. It is the case of commonly diffused recipes fundamental for the local population's diet in Italy, which employ vegetables, legumes, or cereals. The work by Chatzopoulou et al. (2020) highlights that the rediscovery of the Mediterranean Diet by younger generations has nurtured the interest in some specific vegetables (like chicory). In the long run, it will require sustainable management of resources. In the chapter, the authors highlight the marketing opportunities that emerge from the consumption of these products.

Background research provides examples of traditional culinary cultures that have promoted healthy food consumption patterns: in Italy, we can find the case of Apulia Region (Renna et al., 2015) or Sicily which widely employs wild plants in its traditional dishes (Licata et al., 2016).

A strong linkage between local food and culture emerges: the employment of some specific inputs for recipes—inputs that are recognised to give benefits when consumed—characterises not only typical dishes but a diffused knowledge among the local population about the benefits associated with food consumption.

The system of relationships and linkages between places, people, culture, food, and health emerges in Heinrich et al. (2005): local knowledge has represented a stimulus for the diffusion of information about the health benefits of some inputs or ingredients. Local knowledge is passed from one generation to the other: the result is creating a system of traditional food knowledge that associates benefits to plants or food. We can easily imagine how traditional food knowledge, which is part of the heritage of an area or a population, can be a leverage for marketing local food products.

8.4 The relationships between food, tradition, and health

There is no doubt that local populations, especially in rural areas, have a consolidated knowledge of food and plants health attributes. The discovery of some properties of foods has followed emerging insights from traditional culture. There is, then, a solid relationship between food, tradition, and health, a local knowledge about traditional food nurtures that.

The literature provides some impressive cases. The work by Rivera et al. (2005) underlines the relevancy of Mediterranean food plants as a resource for the development of southern Spain. In the work, the authors underline that local plants that can be considered medicinal food plants characterise the local diet in Castilla – La Mancha and Lower Segura Valley.

Another work by Alarcòn et al. (2015) underlines the strong linkage between cultural issues and local heritage's broad employment of food plants.

Heinrich et al. (2005) have studied the implementation of nutraceutical plants in typical food recipes and the diffusion of related knowledge among local populations in the Mediterranean area.

In particular, Heinrich et al. (2005) have described the relationship between local traditions and knowledge flows: "Local traditions rely on information being passed on from one generation to the next in one community or a small region" (p. 6). These considerations are particularly true when applied to rural communities and their food culture that rely on local ingredients and plants.

Italy is rich in local foods, and it is the vibrant essence of the Mediterranean diet. Therefore, as some authors have underlined (Heinrich et al., 2006), the principles of the Mediterranean diet focus on the elements (olive oil, vegetables, etc.) rather than on traditional and local foods.

Italy finds in traditional food knowledge a valuable resource, given the high presence of high-quality typical foods. The number of protected designation of origin (PDO), PGI and traditional guaranteed specialities (TGS) shows that Italy has a consolidated experience in producing not only high-quality food but also in boosting local food production. According to Osservatorio Qualivita, in Italy, there are 656 PDO and 64 TGS that in 2020 made Italy the first country by the number of products in the European Register. This is a strategic asset because it creates business and export opportunities. Therefore, there is a system of knowledge and expertise behind these products that belongs to local and rural communities.

Traditional food knowledge is essential for associating local food consumption with health benefits. Heinrich et al. (2005, 2006) have outlined the abovementioned aspects by adopting an approach based on traditional ecological knowledge (TEK). This knowledge emerges from a group of people who live in a place in close contact with nature. The dynamic aspect of TEK is that it evolves from one generation to the other. The emerging insights from research highlight that starting from what is "good for local people's health" is a good starting point.

In Asia, some health promotion programs for micronutrients are based on the consumption of traditional local food (see, e.g., work by Vuong, 2002 for Vietnam). We can say that policymakers have growing attention to the relationships between nutrition, health, and food systems of indigenous people (Kuhnlein, 2003).

The role of research emerges: research can have a significant role in developing the local food system by underlining the positive benefits associated with traditional food consumption. Therefore, research can reinforce the basis of local traditional food knowledge and provide scientific support to convince good properties that emerge from tradition.

Italy and the central part of Italy provide valuable research insights: we can cite as examples the work by Ranfa et al. (2014, 2015) in Umbria and central Italy, or Piccolo et al. (2020) in Tuscany.

8.5 Analysis

Pulses are the seeds of Leguminosae plants (legumes) consisting of about 750 genera and 19.000 species of herbs, shrubs, trees, and climbers. Legumes as beans (Phaseolus spp.), lentils (Lens culinaris), chickpeas (Cicer arietinum), peas (Pisum spp.), and others are typical crops of the Marche region. They are becoming the "food of the future" both for their nutritional properties and their low environmental impact and sustainability related to agricultural production. In particular, the nutraceutical properties of lentils have been studied in the last years by the University of Camerino through the characterisation of bioactive molecules present in the seeds and the bioactivity of prepared extracts. Among the phytochemicals present in lentils, soyasaponins, belonging to the family of saponins, are triterpenoid glycosides, structurally divided into two groups, one called "A" (bidesmosidic) and the other "B" (monodesmosidic) that possess multiple health-promoting properties, such as lowering of cholesterol (Sagratini et al., 2009, 2013). The quantification of soyasaponins I and βg has been realised by using solid-phase extraction coupled to a liquid chromatography–mass spectrometry (MS) system, showing that soyasaponins I and βg in lentils coming from Visso, Fiastra, Castelluccio di Norcia, Colfiorito were present in concentrations that ranged from 54 to 226 mg/kg and from 436 to 1272 mg/kg, respectively (Vila Donat et al., 2014). In a following paper by the same research group, Micioni Di Bonaventura et al. realised a hydroalcoholic lentil extract (LE) for investigating (1) the hypocholesterolemic action in an animal model by studying the plasma cholesterol level and the concentration of bile acids in the faeces, and (2) the potential prebiotic effect by conducting an in vitro culture fermentation experiment and assessing the level of short-chain fatty acids in the rat faeces. Results showed that LE reduced the plasma cholesterol levels of rats by 16.8% ($P < 0.05$) with an increase of HDL levels ($P > 0.05$) and a decrease of LDL levels ($P > 0.05$). Concerning prebiotic activity, LE showed the same prebiotic ability of inulin and also had a good bifidogenic property by increasing the growth of Bifidobacterium spp in the intestinal microflora (Micioni et al., 2017). Another important class of phytochemicals present in pulses has been studied and characterised, that is, the polyphenolic compounds, using a new HPLC-MS/MS method to quantify 16 of them, that is, gallic acid, catechin, ferulic acid and others. The highest polyphenol levels were found in beans, particularly black beans (459 mg/kg) and ruviotto beans (189 mg/kg); significant levels of polyphenols were also observed in lentils particularly black lentils (137 mg/kg) and quality gold lentils (132 mg/kg). Samples with dark testa (or seed coat), namely black lentils and diavoli beans, had higher antioxidant activity than those with pale testa, and a positive correlation was found between total phenolic content and IC50 (antioxidant activity) for dark-coloured varieties (Giusti et al., 2017, 2018; Caprioli et al., 2018). Giusti et al. (2019) investigated the bioaccessibility of legume polyphenols showing that the cooking process strongly reduces the content in free and bound phenolic compounds and that the processing water is a valuable source of phenolics.

The scientific community now widely recognises that phytonutrients contained in fruit and vegetables, also known as phytochemicals, act as signal molecules by modulating various cellular processes associated with the prevention of various diseases. On this basis, the University of Camerino project on the Mela Rosa dei Monti Sibillini (MR) was aimed to highlight the bioactive components of this ancient apple variety and their health potential. MR is one of the oldest varieties of the Marche region, grown in the foothills between 400 and 900 m of altitude and identifiable for its small size, irregular shape, shades from pink to the purplish-red, intense aroma aromatic, and the sour and sugary flavour (Wandjou et al., 2019). It was recognised as a traditional product of the Marche region in 1998 and as a Slow Food praesidium in 2000. The studies showed that MR and its by-products are an excellent source of phytonutrients such as catechins, B-type proanthocyanidins, triterpene acids, and dihydrochalcones (Wandjou et al., 2020a,b). These substances are endowed with important pharmacological activities such as antioxidant, antitumor, antidiabetic, anti–inflammatory, and neuroprotective. In particular, MR, when compared to other commercial apples, contains higher levels of some of these bioactive compounds (Wandjou et al., 2020b). In two studies, published in Food & Function and

Molecules, it has been shown that hydroalcoholic extracts obtained from MR peel can help in reducing oxidative stress and inflammatory response. These effects were observed in the kidney and liver of rats with induced damage by renal ischemia–reperfusion and carbon tetrachloride, respectively. In particular, the administration of the MR extract significantly reduced the levels of oxidative stress markers such as MDA and MPO, inflammatory cytokines such as TNF-alpha and IL-1, and the expression of NF-kB is an important transcription factor involved in the inflammatory response (Yousefi-Manesh et al., 2019). In the liver, a decrease in the level of transaminases has been observed after the ME extract administration and an increase in the activity of antioxidant enzymes such as superoxide dismutase (Yousefi-Manesh et al., 2020).

In conclusion, these studies showed that MR and their by-products have all the credentials to be used at a nutraceutical level in the formulation of food supplements to prevent diseases related to oxidative stress and inflammation.

Aniseed, Pimpinella anisum, is an annual crop cultivated for centuries in Castignano, a medieval town near Ascoli Piceno, Marche, Italy. This crop mainly was used for its essential oil by local liquor companies until the 1990s when it was replaced by seeds coming from Middle East markets due to globalisation. Its cultivation recovery started recently in the Piceno area,. Scientific research played a pivotal role in promoting its valorisation in the neighbouring territory until the recognition of the Slow Food praesidium in 2017. The research conducted at the University of Camerino on Castignano aniseed showed not only that this ecotype is endowed with a higher essential oil and anethole yields when compared with commercial samples of different geographic origin, but also it contains a higher amount of healthy-promoting compounds such as caffeoylquinic acids and flavonol glycosides, namely apigenin, isoorientin, and luteolin derivatives (Iannarelli et al., 2017). Further studies paved the way for new applications of this crop, especially in the manufacturing of eco-friendly insecticides for crop protection, food commodities, and to combat insect vectors of public health importance (Benelli et al., 2017, 2018; Pavela et al., 2019).

8.6 Discussion and future projects

As outlined in the previous paragraphs, research has highlighted the positive benefits of local food production in the Marche region. At the same time, scholars in business management have explored the importance of

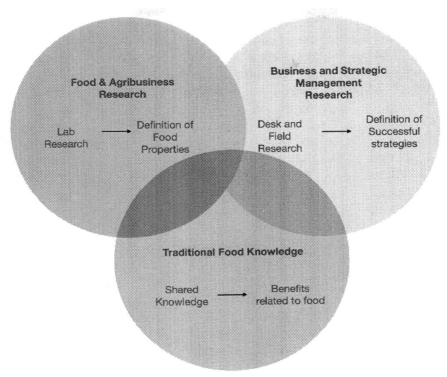

Fig. 8.1 *The three-level of investigation of the problem.*

differentiation strategy for mature industries and have outlined a path for rejuvenating mature products.

We also have outlined that traditional food knowledge can be a source of information about the nutritional properties of food.

As we can understand from this chapter, research can include three different perspectives: one of the marketers and strategic marketing specialists, one of the agrifood researchers, and then one of the local populations.

From the dialogue between those three areas, research activity emerges (Fig. 8.1) whose aims are:

1. to support with science-based evidence, the traditional food knowledge diffused among the local population;
2. to build differentiation strategies upon reliable and trustable elements that emerge from research carried in labs by agrifood researchers; and
3. to support the system of traditional food knowledge.

Adopting a bottom–up approach in research on nutraceuticals that evaluates emerging information from local populations and tests them could also be leverage for researchers who want to interact with local producers.

Some interesting research questions emerge and could be at the centre of future research projects:

– how to successfully communicate healthy food properties to consumers?

– what is the role of traditional food knowledge in making information more reliable and accessible to consumers?

– how to strategically employ tradition to extend the product life cycle and improve its competitiveness over time?

From the chapter, it also emerges the proactive role of Slow Food Association: the recognition of a slow food presidium in 2017 was a further asset for local producers and it gives new opportunities for the development of the production. Therefore, once there is recognition of the typical traits of a product and its quality, information that science provides in terms of nutritional components can help in the development of local production. In this specific case, slow food could facilitate knowledge transmission from researchers to producers and consumers, making information more accessible and helping producers and consumers to maintain a comprehensive approach to quality, that also includes health issues.

8.7 Conclusions

This chapter provides an overview of the relationships between traditional products, local knowledge, and health benefits: emerging insights from research underline the potential benefits of local food consumption due to the recognised properties and features of the examined foods.

The described scenario opens new perspectives for businesses whose margins are generally limited.

Farmers seek differentiation elements, and in a country that is overcrowded in terms of quality and local products, as we have seen, the inner nutritional properties of food can represent strategic leverage for creating a competitive advantage.

We can say that the combination of tradition, local food culture, typical products, and healthy benefits can be extremely useful for marketing and rejuvenating mature products.

Therefore, the relationship between local production and research is crucial: food researchers can help to validate the properties of functional local products and confirm the traditional food knowledge diffused among rural communities. Researchers in marketing and strategic management can help farmers develop effective management of the product and help revitalise mature businesses.

Another exciting aspect is that this approach nurtures a sense of alignment between researchers and farmers: researchers, when adopting a bottom-up approach in the definition of their object of study, give credits to widespread local knowledge and valorise what emerges from traditional food culture. This contributes to bridging the gap between professionals and academics and reducing the distance between thinkers and doers (Cavicchi et al. 2014; Santini et al., 2016).

References

Alarcón, R., Pardo-de-Santayana, M., Priestley, C., Morales, R., Heinrich, M., 2015. Medicinal and local food plants in the south of Alava (Basque Country, Spain). J. Ethnopharmacol. 176, 207–224.

Aleffi, C., Cavicchi, A., 2021. The role of food and culinary heritage for postdisaster recovery: the case of earthquake in the Marche Region (Italy). Journal of Gastronomy and Tourism 4, 113–128.

Anderson, C.R., Zeithaml, C.P., 1984. Stage of the product life cycle, business strategy, and business performance. Acad. Manag. J. 27 (1), 5–24.

Andrews, J., Smith, D.C., 1996. In search of the marketing imagination: factors affecting the creativity of marketing programs for mature products. Journal of Marketing Research 33 (2), 174–187.

Basu, S.K., Thomas, J.E., Acharya, S.N., 2007. Prospects for growth in global nutraceutical and functional food markets: a Canadian perspective. Aust. J. Basic Appl. Sci. 1 (4), 637–649.

Benelli, G., Pavela, R., Iannarelli, R., Petrelli, R., Cappellacci, L., Cianfaglione, K., Afshar, F.H., Nicoletti, M., Canale, A., Maggi, F., 2017. Synergized mixtures of Apiaceae essential oils and related plant-borne compounds: larvicidal effectiveness on the filariasis vector Culex quinquefasciatus Say. Ind. Crops Prod. 96, 186–195.

Benelli, G., Pavela, R., Petrelli, R., Cappellacci, L., Canale, A., Senthil-Nathan, S., Maggi, F., 2018. Not just popular spices! Essential oils from Cuminum cyminum and Pimpinella anisum are toxic to insect pests and vectors without affecting non-target invertebrates. Ind. Crops Prod. 124, 236–243.

Bonanno, A., 2013. Functional foods as differentiated products: the Italian Yogurt Market. European Review of Agricultural Economics 40 (1), 45–71.

Bröring, S., Martin Cloutier, L., Leker, J., 2006. The front end of innovation in an era of industry convergence: evidence from nutraceuticals and functional foods. R&D Management 36 (5), 487–498.

Cappelletti, R., Mezzetti, B., Balducci, F., Diamanti, J., Capocasa, F., 2013. Morphological, nutraceutical and chemical characterisation of globe artichoke (Cynara Cardunculus L. Var. Scolymus (L.) Landraces typically cultivated in Marche area. Acta Hortic 983, 3.

Caprioli, G., Nzekoue, F.K., Giusti, F., Vittori, S., Sagratini, G., 2018. Optimisation of an extraction method for the simultaneous quantification of sixteen polyphenols in thirty-one pulse samples by using HPLC-MS/MS dynamic-MRM triple quadrupole. Food Chem. 266, 490–497.

Cavicchi, A., Santini, C., Bailetti, L., 2014. Mind the "academician-practitioner" gap: an experience-based model in the food and beverage sector. Qualitative Market Research: An International Journal 17 (4), 319–335.

Chatzopoulou, E., Carocho, M., Di Gioia, F., Petropoulos, S.A., 2020. The beneficial health effects of vegetables and wild edible greens: the case of the mediterranean diet and its sustainability. Applied Sciences 10 (24), 9144.

Costa, A.I.A., Jongen, W.M.F., 2006. New insights into consumer-led food product development. Trends Food Sci. Technol. 17 (8), 457–465.

Cutler, H., Ozawa, T., 2007. The dynamics of the "Mature" product cycle and market reycling, flying-geese style: an empirical examination and policy implications. Contemporary Economic Policy 25 (1), 67–78.

Giusti, F., Caprioli, G., Ricciutelli, M., Torregiani, E., Vittori, S., Sagratini, G., 2018. Analysis of 17 polyphenolic compounds in organic and conventional legumes by high-performance liquid chromatography-diode array detection (HPLC-DAD) and evaluation of their antioxidant activity. Int. J. Food Sci. Nutr. 69 (5), 557–565.

Giusti, F., Caprioli, G., Ricciutelli, M., Vittori, S., Sagratini, G., 2017. Determination of fourteen polyphenols in pulses by high performance liquid chromatography-diode array detection (HPLC-DAD) and correlation study with antioxidant activity and colour. Food Chem. 221, 689–697.

Giusti, F., Capuano, E., Sagratini, G., Pellegrini, N., 2019. Comprehensive investigation of the behavior of phenolic compounds in legumes during domestic cooking and in vitro digestion. Food Chem. 285, 458–467.

Goldberg, I., 2012. Functional foods: designer foods, pharmafoods, nutraceuticals. Springer Science & Business Media, Germany.

Gul, K., Singh, A.K., Jabeen, R., 2016. Nutraceuticals and functional foods: the foods for the future world. Crit. Rev. Food Sci. Nutr. 56 (16), 2617–2627.

Heinrich, M., Leonti, M., Nebel, S., Peschel, W., 2005. "Local food-nutraceuticals": an example of a multidisciplinary research project on local knowledge. Journal of Physiology and Pharmacology. Supplement 56 (1), 5–22.

Heinrich, M., Müller, W.E., Galli, C., 2006. Local Mediterranean Food Plants and Nutraceuticals Vol. 59. Karger Medical and Scientific Publishers.

Iannarelli, R., Caprioli, G., Sut, S., Dall'Acqua, S., Fiorini, D., Vittori, S., Maggi, F., 2017. Valorizing Overlooked local crops in the era of globalization: the case of aniseed (Pimpinella anisum L.) from Castignano (central Italy). Industrial Crops & Products 104, 99–110.

J. van buul, V., Brouns, F.J, 2015. Nutrition and health claims as marketing tools. Crit. Rev. Food Sci. Nutr. 55 (11), 1552–1560.

Jiménez-Morales, M., Blasco, M.M., 2021. Presence and strategic use of the Mediterranean Diet in food marketing: Analysis and association of nutritional values and advertising claims from 2011 to 2020. NFS Journal 24, 1–6.

Kuhnlein, H.V., 2003. Micronutrient nutrition and traditional food systems of indigenous peoples. Food Nutrition and agriculture 32, 33–39.

Licata, M., Tuttolomondo, T., Leto, C., Virga, G., Bonsangue, G., Cammalleri, I...., La Bella, S., 2016. A survey of wild plant species for food use in Sicily (Italy)–results of a 3-year study in four regional parks. J. Ethnobiol. Ethnomed. 12 (1), 1–24.

Lucchetti, L., Zitti, S., Taffetani, F., 2019. Ethnobotanical uses in the Ancona district (Marche region, Central Italy). J. Ethnobiol. Ethnomed. 15 (9), 1–33.

Micioni Di Bonaventura, M.V., Cecchini, C., Vila-Donat, P., Caprioli, G., Cifani, C., Coman, M.M., Cresci, A., Fiorini, D., Ricciutelli, M., Silvi, S., Vittori, S., Sagratini, G., 2017. Evaluation of the hypocholesterolemic effect and prebiotic activity of a lentil (Lens culinaris Medik) extract. Molecular Nutrition and Food Research, 61(11), 1700403.

Morresi, C., Cianfruglia, L., Armeni, T., Mancini, F., Tenore, G., D'Urso, E., Micheletti, A., Ferretti, G., Bacchetti, T., 2018. Polyphenolic compounds and nutraceutical properties of old and new apple cultivars. J. Food Biochem. 42, e12641.

Nasri, H., Baradaran, A., Shirzad, H., Rafieian-Kopaei, M., 2014. New concepts in nutraceu-ticals as alternative for pharmaceuticals. International Journal of Preventive Medicine 5 (12), 1487.

Naylor, R.W., Droms, C.M., Haws, K.L., 2009. Eating with a purpose: Consumer response to functional food health claims in conflicting versus complementary information envi-ronments. Journal of Public Policy & Marketing 28 (2), 221–233.

Pavela, R., Benelli, G., Pavoni, L., Bonacucina, G., Cespi, M., Cianfaglione, K., Bajalan, I., Morshedloo, M.R., Lupidi, G., Romano, D., Canale, A., Maggi, F., 2019. Microemulsions for delivery of Apiaceae essential oils—towards highly effective and eco-friendly mos-quito larvicides? Ind. Crops Prod. 129, 631–640.

Piccolo, E.L., Landi, M., Ceccanti, C., Mininni, A.N., Marchetti, L., Massai, R.…, Remorini, D., 2020. Nutritional and nutraceutical properties of raw and traditionally obtained flour from chestnut fruit grown in Tuscany. Eur. Food Res. Technol. 246 (9), 1867–1876.

Ranfa, A., Maurizi, A., Romano, B., Bodesmo, M., 2014. The importance of traditional uses and nutraceutical aspects of some edible wild plants in human nutrition: the case of Umbria (central Italy). Plant Biosystems-An International Journal Dealing with all Aspects of Plant Biology 148 (2), 297–306.

Ranfa, A., Orlandi, F., Maurizi, A., Bodesmo, M., 2015. Ethnobotanical knowledge and nutritional properties of two edible wild plants from Central Italy: Tordylium apulum L. and Urospermum dalechampii (L.) FW Schmid. Journal of Applied Botany and Food Quality 88 (1), 249–254.

Renna, M., Rinaldi, V.A., Gonnella, M., 2015. The Mediterranean Diet between traditional foods and human health: the culinary example of Puglia (Southern Italy). International Journal of Gastronomy and Food Science 2 (2), 63–71.

Rivera, D., Obon, C., Inocencio, C., Heinrich, M., Verde, A., Fajardo, J., Llorach, R., 2005. The ethnobotanical study of local Mediterranean food plants as medicinal resources in Southern Spain. J Physiol Pharmacol 56 (Suppl 1), 97–114.

Sagratini, G., Caprioli, G., Maggi, F., Font, G., Giardinà, D., Mañes, J., Meca, G., Ricciutelli, M., Sirocchi, V., Torregiani, E., Vittori, S., 2013. Determination of Soyasaponins I and βg in Raw and Cooked Legumes by Solid Phase Extraction (SPE) coupled to liquid chromatography (LC)−mass spectrometry (MS) and assessment of their bioaccessibility by an in vitro digestion model. J. Agric. Food Chem. 61, 1702–1709.

Sagratini, G., Zuo, Y., Caprioli, G., Cristalli, G., Giardinà, D., Maggi, F., Molin, L., Ricciutelli, M., Traldi, P., Vittori, S., 2009. Quantification of Soyasaponins I and VI in Italian Lentil seeds by solid phase extraction (SPE) and high performance liquid chromatography-mass spectrometry (HPLC-MS). J. Agric. Food Chem. 57, 11226–11233.

Santini, C., Marinelli, E., Boden, M., Cavicchi, A., Haegeman, K., 2016. Reducing the dis-tance between thinkers and doers in the entrepreneurial discovery process: an explor-atory study. Journal of Business Research 69 (5), 1840–1844.

Sarkar, S., Costa, A.I., 2008. Dynamics of open innovation in the food industry. Trends Food Sci. Technol. 19 (11), 574–580.

Sujarwo, W., Arinasa, I.B.K., Salomone, F., Caneva, G., Fattorini, S., 2014. Cultural erosion of Balinese indigenous knowledge of food and nutraceutical plants. Economic Botany 68 (4), 426–437.

Vila Donat, P., Caprioli, G., Conti, P., Maggi, F., Ricciutelli, M., Torregiani, E., Vittori, S., Sagratini, G., 2014. Rapid quantification of Soyasaponins I and βg in Italian Lentils by high-performance liquid chromatography (HPLC)−tandem mass spectrometry (MS/MS). Food Anal. Methods 7, 1024–1031.

Vuong, L.T., 2002. Underutilised ß-carotene-rich crops of Vietnam. Food Nutr. Bull. 21 (2), 173–181.

Wandjou, J.G.N., Sut, S., Giuliani, C., Fico, G., Papa, F., Ferraro, S., Caprioli, G., Maggi, F., Dall'Acqua, S., 2019. Characterization of nutrients, polyphenols and volatile compo-nents of the ancient apple cultivar 'Mela Rosa Dei Monti Sibillini' from Marche region, central Italy. Int. J. Food Sci. Nutr. 70 (7), 796–812.

Wandjou, J.G.N., Mevi, S., Sagratini, G., Vittori, S., Dall'Acqua, S., Caprioli, G., Lupidi, G., Mombelli, G., Arpini, S., Allegrini, P., Les, F., López, V., Maggi, F., 2020a. Antioxidant and enzyme inhibitory properties of the polyphenolic-rich extract from an ancient apple variety of Central Italy (Mela Rosa dei Monti Sibillini). Plants 9, 9.

Wandjou, J.G.N., Lancioni, L., Barbalace, M.C., Hrelia, S., Papa, F., Sagratini, G., Vittori, S., Dall'Acqua, S., Caprioli, G., Beghelli, D., Angeloni, C., Lupidi, G., Maggi, F., 2020b. Comprehensive characterization of phytochemicals and biological activities of the Italian ancient apple 'Mela Rosa dei Monti Sibillini. Food Res. Int. 137, 109422.

Yousefi-Manesh, H., Hemmati, S., Shirooie, S., Nabavi, S.M., Bonakdar, A.T., Fayaznia, R., Asgardoon, M.H., Dehnavi, A.Z., Ghafouri, M., Wandjou, J.G.N., Caprioli, C., Sut, S., Maggi, F., Dall'Acqua, S., 2019. Protective effects of hydroalcoholic extracts from an ancient apple variety 'Mela Rosa dei Monti Sibillini' against renal ischemia/reperfusion injury in rats. Food & Function 10 (11), 7544–7552.

Yousefi-Manesh, H., Dehpour, A.R., Ansari-Nasab, S., Hemmati, S., Sadeghi, M.A., Shahraki, R.H., Shirooie, S., Nabavi, S.M., Wandjou, J.G.N., Sut, S., Caprioli, G., Dall'Acqua, S., Maggi, F., 2020. Hepatoprotective Effects of Standardized Extracts from an Ancient Italian Apple Variety (Mela Rosa dei Monti Sibillini) against Carbon Tetrachloride (CCl4)-Induced Hepatotoxicity in Rats. Molecules 25 (8), 1816.

CHAPTER 9

Organic and Made in Tuscany Spirulina: the story of Severino Becagli

Cristina Santini[a], Alessio Cavicchi[b]

[a]University San Raffaele Rome, Italy
[b]Department of Agriculture, Food and Environment, University of Pisa, Pisa, Italy

9.1 Introduction

The Spirulina market is extremely dynamic worldwide: the degree of competition is growing due to the emerging of low-cost producers from China and India. Competitive borders are blurring in nutraceuticals, and Spirulina has multiple employment with different margin structures and profitability changes according to the type of final output. New entrants, even players from other industries, are reshaping the business. This chapter explores the case of Severino Becagli, a young company that operates in the South of Tuscany and produces organic Spirulina. The company releases on the market different types of products, from powder spirulina to food products containing Spirulina. The company markets to consumers organic made in Tuscany Spirulina and seeks to differentiate its production by combining together organic principles with the country of origin. Thus, this chapter aims to answer the following research question: how to improve competitive advantage by using country of origin in the Spirulina market? The chapter is structured as follows: in the next paragraph, we provide an analysis of the world market and then of the Italian one. Furthermore, an analysis of challenges with a specific focus on costs and management problems is outlined. Finally, after having introduced the business, we describe the case study and then we draw some final remarks.

9.2 Market

Spirulina is a microalga that represents an attractive and booming market. It is often called "the food of the future" because it is rich in health benefits and is considered a sustainable product.

Case Studies on the Business of Nutraceuticals, Functional and Super Foods
DOI: https://doi.org/10.1016/B978-0-12-821408-4.00004-3
161

The global market for Spirulina in 2021 was worth 348 million USD and, with an average CAAGR of 15%, it will probably reach 779 million USD by 2026 (Source: market data forecast). Estimations about the size of the market differ according to the source: some news declares that the global dimension of the market in 2025 will reach 629.26 million USD (global news wire). After COVID, it is hard to have precise forecasts; in any case, all the available sources of information agree in defining the market as growing and promising.

The market for Spirulina can be divided into different product types; according to insights from Enzing et al. (2014), we can segment the market into two mainstreams: the dried alga, which can be sold as a dietary supplement, and the extract of the alga that can be added to food to create superfoods.

There are many reasons behind the global growth of Spirulina. First of all, consumers seek novel foods and nutraceuticals. In general, foods with healthy properties attract consumers. Research on consumers' acceptance of functional foods and nutraceuticals aims to define the profile of consumers who buy nutraceuticals and superfoods: from this research stream, it emerges how, besides differences at the country level, consumers who are firmly convinced about the importance of a healthy lifestyle are oriented to try novel foods and to introduce them into their diets (Moons et al., 2017).

Thus, Spirulina has encountered a breeding ground for its diffusion due to consumers' interest and the characteristics of this product have stimulated a booming demand.

In fact, Spirulina represents a very nutritious ingredient: the high presence of vitamins and proteins, antioxidants, pigments and minerals, among others, motivate the interest shown by the feed and the food industries.

Institutions and governments have stimulated the production of this product: in Europe, the European Commission has dedicated much attention to the production of algae and Spirulina (Enzing et al., 2014).

Many countries have seen in Spirulina an answer for facing the food crisis due to its richness in nutritional components. For example, in Zambia, the government has tried to support the development of Spirulina to enrich food and to provide dietary supplements for those population groups who are suffering from food scarcity and nutritional problems.

The growing concern for the climate status of the planet supports algae production: Europe is committed to promoting the principles of circular economy and to developing the farm to fork strategy (EC 2012, 2018, 2020a, Enzing, 2014; EC 2020b), and Spirulina perfectly fits with this scenario, since it has a minimal carbon footprint. It can play a key role in the formulation of meat substitutes.

As previously observed, it is tough to find specific information about the Spirulina market and production: background research underlines how fragmented the industry is and how difficult it is to gain a precise overview of market trends and dynamics (Thomas et al., 2020).

According to Araújo (2021), in Europe, 225 companies produce macroalgae (67%) and microalgae (33%); out of the 225, there are 222 Spirulina producers spread among 23 countries. The leading producers in Europe are Spain, France, Ireland, Norway, UK, Germany, and Portugal. From the study, we can have a general idea of the producers' profile: most companies were established in the last decade, and production mainly employs ponds (83% vs 17% photobioreactors). The production sites are still small-scale. According to Araùjo (2021), 19 Italian companies produce Spirulina, and most of them are located in Northern Italy; nevertheless, there are no official statistical sources to validate this information.

The implementation of micro- and macro-algae is multiple: it can range from human food, cosmetics and wellbeing, food supplements, feed to pharmaceuticals or biofuels.

According to the European Economic and Social Committee, the Spirulina is part of the Blue Bio-Economy system: "The blue bio-economy means economic activities and value creation based on sustainable and smart use of renewable aquatic resources and the related expertise" (European Economic and Social Committee, 2019). This sector is estimated to generate 5.4 million jobs, actively contributing to national economic growth. European Union has designed a Blue Growth Strategy, and some countries in Europe have reshaped their national research policies to include specific resources for this sector.

Defining where research is going and how it is supported is extremely difficult: Spirulina can be sold under different "shapes" (powders, extract, etc.) and can be employed in many ways for various purposes. Therefore, the scenario of stakeholders interested in Spirulina is vast. It includes agri-food, nutraceutical, cosmeceutical companies, and companies that operate in the green industry, such as the green energy sector.

Innovation insights can emerge from a cross-collaboration among companies operating in different fields, and the business borders are blurring, so competition is spread among various industries. The multiple sources of innovation create a very dynamic environment, although some difficulties emerge in Europe: as for the algae production industry, there are a series of technological, regulatory, and market-related barriers that limit the sector's development (Ruiz et al., 2016). Thus, it is a promising sector with a considerable potential for sustainable development, although there is still so much to gain in knowledge and innovation. According to Rahman (2020), the European spirulina business has to face many challenges for improving the marketing of microalgae products: biomass production cost, technical breakthroughs, access to venture capital, and academic and industrial training.

9.3 Italy

In Italy, the business of Spirulina is growing. As we have previously outlined, it is difficult to estimate the number of Spirulina producers with precision. Some information can emerge from associations that collect producers by production features, such as the type of production (organic, for example).

In particular, from preliminary web-based research, we have found an association, the USBI, l'Unione Spirulina Biologica Italiana (Association of Italian organic spirulina producers) that provides some numbers about the sector.

Table 9.1 shows the detailed list of companies in the association.

Table 9.1 USBI details.

Name	URL	Description	Producers/companies	Websites
Unione Spirulina Biologica Italiana	https://unionespirulina.it/	Unione Italiana produttori di alga spirulina Biologica	Azienda Agricola Salera	http://salera.net
			Azienda Agricola Prato della Voja	https://www.pratodellavoja.it
			Azienda Agricola Reggiani Giuseppe—Farmodena	https://www.farmodena.it/azienda
			Azienda Agricola Zotta Natalino	http://www.zoc-canatalino.com
			Azienda Agricola Bosello - Alghessere	https://www.alghessere.it
			Azienda Sabar	https://www.sabar.it
			Azienda Agricola Mauro Comasco	http://www.comascofiori.it

The yearly average production of the Association is 5–7 tons of Spirulina with an estimated value of 500.000 euros. The main competitors are organic producers from India and China, with lower production costs. One of the main differences of the Italian grown Spirulina compared to Indian and Chinese ones is the taste: Chinese or Indian Spirulina has a more pungent taste, according to USBI.

We must underline that background research is rich in studies that explore the role of spirulina taste in the formulation of novel foods. Still, it lacks studies investigating the role of country of origin on the taste of Spirulina.

USBI has become the exclusive spirulina supplier of Il Nuovo Fresco, a company with more than 25 years of experience in the agrifood sector, to produce functional foods (pasta, drink, snacks, pesto, and other products). Another example of partnership is the one between Andriani, a company that is specialised in the production of gluten-free pasta, and ApuliaKundi, the leading spirulina producers in the Apulia region (South Italy).

Italian researchers are now focusing on two significant issues: the first challenge is improving knowledge of spirulina cultivation; the second challenge is highlighting new ways for employing this input. The business's profitability has progressively attracted, as previously outlined, new players from other industries. New entrants have intensified the number of potential entrants and brought in the business new knowledge and technology.

One example is Tolo Green, a company initially in the energy sector whose core business was photovoltaics. They have combined photovoltaics with greenhouses and, for the Dubai Expo, Tologreen has created a system that converts carbon dioxide produced by visitors of the pavilion and creates an environment that "breathes through the energy produced by the Spirulina Algae" and it promotes wellbeing. The above-described example shows how companies exploit expertise gained in different businesses (in this case, green energy) to develop spirulina plants.

From the collaboration with scientific researchers, other opportunities have emerged for Spirulina. Researchers have investigated how to produce spirulina algae by employing geothermal energy in Chiusdino (https://www.thinkgeoenergy.com/cultivating-geothermal-and-spirulina-creates-100-jobs-in-tuscany-italy/). Other researches are focusing on photobioreactors and the replacement of natural light with led light. Some projects explore how to recycle the waste from olive oil production in microalgae production plants.

The provided examples underline that there is so much going on in this field, and research aims to provide solutions for keeping costs under control and improving spirulina plants' productivity.

9.4 Costs, margins, and value chains

We must underline that the business's profitability changes according to the finished product sold to the market since margins are different.

According to researchers (in particular, Voort et al., 2015), algae products are classified into three types of products following their market value: high-, medium-, and low-value products. High-value products have a lower volume, and their target is personal care and pharmaceuticals. Instead, low-value products are available in larger quantities and are employed in the energy and bioremediation businesses. Medium value products are addressed to food, feed, and chemicals and materials businesses.

Rahman (2020) explores the value chain of algae products and provides some insights for understanding the process of value creation: the value of the product depends on its composition (in particular concentration and amount of some "properties"), application, and formulation (granular, powder, and so forth). Finished products have a considerable variability of their value. According to the Eaba (European Algae Biomass Association), the value of some pigments (such as the fucoxanthin, which is available in some multicellular brown algae) is around 45.000 USD per kilo.

Following some specific studies (Ruiz et al. 2016), pigments gain a higher market price, especially in the cosmetics, healthcare, and food additives segments. The biofuel industry has the lowest market price for algae producers, followed by the food-feed industry; the two businesses where producers can gain higher market prices are the ones of food additives and cosmetics healthcare.

The growing demand and the possibility of gaining high profits increase the appeal of Spirulina and microalgae in general. However, as it emerges from Caporgno and Marhys (2018), drawbacks emerge when discussing large-scale commercialisation of microalgae-based products: today, the challenge is working to improve the efficiency of large-scale facilities. Meanwhile, producers have to find ways to maximise their profits and margins, given a scenario characterised by growing demand and fierce competition emerging from Chinese producers who can realise mass production.

9.5 Case of Spirulina Becagli

9.5.1 Story

The Severino Becagli is a newborn company that produces organic Spirulina near Grosseto, in Southern Tuscany. It is a start-up company, launched by Tommaso Becagli, a young entrepreneur whose family name (Becagli) is famous in Tuscany due to the prolonged activity of the family in the fabric production in the city of Prato (Northern Tuscany).

Severino Becagli was Tommaso Becagli's great-grandfather; the idea behind the choice of the company name was to recall the story of the family and highlight the role of tradition. Company location underlines the importance of tradition: the company has its headquarter in a traditional country house that dates back to the 19th century. The company is young from all the points of view: the average age of employees is less than 45 years old.

In 1986, the Becagli family established production of grain stocks on a surface of 500 hectares in the province of Grosseto. It was around 2009 when they have jumped into the biogas business, and they soon had to manage the problem of nitrogen emerging from the production process. This has represented the sparkle for an interest in microalgae: algae represented a viable solution for facing the problem of wastes and nitrogen. Given the opportunities arising from the market, the company has decided to dedicate its attention to Spirulina.

Tommaso Becagli says "we were standing at a crossroad: on one side we had a superfood and the food of the next future; on the other side we had traditional cultivations. We had to choose a 2.0 product for being in line with the times".

The company's mission is to reach as many persons as possible, although some people may consider Spirulina an elite product. This product is relatively new to the market, and the price is high: "the global market in 2018 has generated a turnover of 346 million USD in 2018, and the Financial Times estimates that it will reach 779 million USD by 2023. 3/4 of the total turnover comes from Asia and producers have lower production costs than ours".

9.5.2 Differentiation strategy

Spirulina can be a leverage for promoting products: "Spirulina became a claim on the labels: although sometimes the percentage in the product is extremely low, companies mention it for improving sales. This emerges in pet food, for example".

As a claim, the implementation of the brand-name Spirulina introduces the need for companies to differentiate further: not all the produced Spirulina are the same.

"We are committed to informing about the production of our Spirulina. We produce organic Spirulina, but we are afraid that our product can be perceived as similar to others with an organic 'label', but they are not".

A challenge is the reliability of organic labels for Spirulina: the ongoing competition emerging from Chinese producers increases a debate about the price since their output is less expensive than the European one.

Severino Becagli has decided to build its uniqueness on the synergy of two issues: being organic and made in Tuscany: "we can face the request for lowering the price only by offering a high-quality organic and made in Tuscany product. We have to market our product as a made in Tuscany product: we are settled in a wonderful place, and we sell wellbeing and beauty".

The idea of promoting an organic made in Tuscany Spirulina gives a new light to the issue of competitiveness in this dynamic industry. Algae, in general, are not associated with a place of production; wakame is the only exception since it is famous for being a Japanese alga, although we can find production sites even outside Japan. Therefore, to employ a country of origin for marketing a product and realising a differentiation strategy, in this specific case, is challenging. Severino Becagli wants to promote a Made in Tuscany concept that highlights a story of tradition and commitment to realise quality products. The idea behind the made in Tuscany organic Spirulina is to produce in a safe and beautiful environment by respecting and preserving natural resources. The company makes a further step: they create a link between Spirulina, country of origin, and food by producing food products enriched with Spirulina with inputs that are locally produced.

9.5.3 Business and the product portfolio

The Severino Becagli company operates in different segments (Fig. 9.1): it covers the food, nutraceuticals (providing fresh, extract and powder Spirulina), and beauty businesses.

The company sells its products directly and indirectly. Direct sales happen through the point of sales at the factory or through the web: different

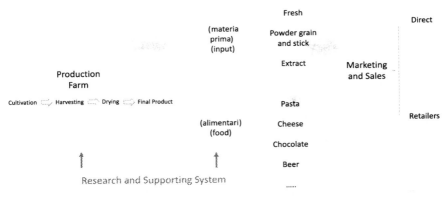

Fig. 9.1 *Business.*

sizes and product formats are available, and the company has developed some packaging solutions that can facilitate the daily intake of Spirulina.

Together with "materia prima" (raw material), as they call it, or powder grain and sticks of Spirulina, which represents a considerable share of their revenues, the company sells food added with Spirulina.

The role of research is relevant in the company.

Besides all the research insights applied in the management of the production plan, research insights are employed to efficiently perform market uptakes.

Research provides information about the composition of the algae. Some research processes are also linked to the presence of certification (organic and kosher, for example) in the company.

Behind the marketability of food products, there is broad research carried out for assessing product formulation and product acceptance.

"We provide a product that has got health benefits for a cost that goes around 50 euros per month (average price for a Spirulina powder for 1 month of intake). It is not easy to communicate to people that spending money for their health is acceptable: people tend to purchase what is prescribed by doctors, but in this case, we have to inform, educate and motivate people to buy spirulina".

There is no doubt that selling food products represents a leverage for improving knowledge about Spirulina, and it is also the sector where, as we have seen before, the margin is higher.

There is a critical issue concerning this point that emerges from the interview: "When we give people the pasta with the Spirulina, we eliminate the problem of understanding how to intake Spirulina: everything is ready, so the consumer only has to purchase it. We have created some outstanding products. For example, we have performed many consumers tests before releasing our version of mayonnaise. Our idea was to employ everyday products that people normally eat (like pasta, mayonnaise, chocolate) to introduce a new ingredient—Spirulina—in people's lives. The real point is about the percentage of Spirulina, which is not as high in some products to bring a real benefit".

Creating a superfood with Spirulina is a way for stimulating curiosity about the product and will facilitate the intake of Spirulina by powder or sticks.

Background research confirms the validity of this idea: as outlined by Raudenbush and Frank (1999), having a familiarity with a type of food could reduce the neophobia towards some ingredients. According to some researchers (Pliner and Hobden, 1992), neophobia is a phenomenon that frequently happens when consumers meet novel foods: it induces a reluctance to eat unfamiliar foods. In light of the elements mentioned above, pasta or everyday food are tools for educating consumers about Spirulina and reducing neophobia.

This is an exciting point of view because, on one side, it is clear the company's mission to inform about the benefits of this alga; on the other, Spirulina added products become relevant for marketing reasons and for gaining profits.

This company has put efforts in the formulation of superfood products: they have selected producing companies for cooperating with them in the definition of a product portfolio to be marketed under the label "Severino Becagli". They have defined the optimum content of Spirulina for meeting consumers' expectations, and they have then worked on the communication campaign and strategy to overcome the resistance to the green colour.

Background research shows that the investigation of consumer orientation is a key resource in developing novel foods (Moskowitz and Hartmann, 2008). Grahl et al. (2018) provide a detailed overview of how consumer science and sensory analysis can be employed to formulate Spirulina-based novel foods. It also highlights that Spirulina novel foods and Spirulina, in general, are associated with three aspects that can be considered strategic marketing leverages: innovativeness, healthiness, and sustainability.

In light of these evidence, it is entirely motivated the decision of Severino Becagli to highlight its organic orientation.

9.6 Final remarks and open questions

The Story of Severino Becagli is successful: it narrates about a young company that has introduced a new product in the hearth of Tuscany, and it aims to bring a novel, healthy and innovative food. This story is also paradigmatic for understanding the challenges that spirulina start-ups must face. This case study introduces the reading to reflect upon the sustainability of a firm's competitive advantage in the long run.

Spirulina has excellent market potential since it has many applications, and consumers' awareness grows. The production system and the process of margin definition open to many business solutions: we have seen that research provides insights for helping companies formulate novel foods. We observe another interesting phenomenon: the predominant attention towards efficacy in production and the entrants of new industry players. Many companies are operating in the energy sector, putting their expertise at the service of spirulina producers. New business companies embrace the principles of circular economy and sustainability: in some cases, green energy operators fund the production of Spirulina. The emerging concept is that Spirulina is fast-moving to become a 100% sustainable produced output.

In the above-described scenario, new challenges emerge for the Severino Becagli company: What role is the "made in Tuscany" brand? What is the role of organic certification? These two questions introduce another question: How to differentiate its production? Given the rapid changes in the competitive environment, the entrance of new players, and the structure of margins in the industry, the company needs to highlight an effective differentiation strategy. At the same time, it becomes more and more important where the company wants to operate: what will be the future of the food business unit? How many efforts and resources should the company invest in producing food products? Will it integrate the production, or will it outsource food production entirely and create a partnership with other companies? The decision about the company's vertical integration could be an additional source of differentiation: it would trace a new development trajectory for Spirulina-based companies.

The diffusion of technology is a critical issue in the development of the spirulina business: technology is progressively reshaping the industry. We have seen how it contributes to the reshaping of productive systems by promoting a circular economy approach when defining business models. Thus, technology is opening new market possibilities for Spirulina. Some companies are developing small–scale plants solution; this will further fragment the production of Spirulina on one side, and on the other, will make spirulina production accessible and capable of being integrated into small companies organisational production.

The concept of small–scale production makes a further step up to conceive home production sites for Spirulina. The solution proposed by Photo Syntetica, a brand of the UK EcoLogicStudio Ltd goes in this direction: the project's mission is to introduce high–tech cultivation in everyday life (from the website). The output of the process is a solution for cultivating Spirulina in people's homes. What is extremely interesting is the approach of the founders of the company. They start from original exploitation of microalga for interior design: microalgae are elements with a biologic intelligence that can interact with the technological systems available in the architecture of a building.

Other companies are selling Photobioreactors for domestic production of Spirulina: it is the case of Algaelab. Similar solutions were supported by EU projects, as in the case of Brevel.

From this discussion, it emerges that the business of Spirulina is hugely dynamic; for start-up companies, it is hard to define a winning strategy in the long run.

Elements of product uniqueness derived from the location could help maintain a competitive advantage in the long run.

In a competitive scenario where borders are blurring and where there are diverging trends (see, e.g., small scale solutions vs large scales; health benefits vs novel food with limited contents of Spirulina), it could be an advantage being settled in a place, Tuscany, that makes it possible to exploit the "country of origin" brand. Probably one way could be the promotion of "made in Tuscany" novel food products inspired by a 0KM/Food Miles philosophy, but this is, again, something new in the business. In this case, Consumer Science and research could be pivotal for providing information.

Acknowledgements

We would like to thank Tommaso Becagli, Leonardo Berni, and the Staff of the Severino Becagli Company for sharing their story and for their support.

References

Araújo, R., Vázquez Calderón, F., Sánchez López, J., Azevedo, I.C., Bruhn, A., Fluch, S...., Ullmann, J., 2021. Current status of the algae production industry in Europe: an emerging sector of the Blue Bioeconomy. Front. Marine Sci. 7, 1247.

Caporgno, M.P., Mathys, A., 2018. Trends in microalgae incorporation into innovative food products with potential health benefits. Front. Nutr. 5, 58.

EC (2012). Commission Communication COM/2012/494. Blue growth opportunities for marine and maritime sustainable growth. https://ec.europa.eu/maritimeaffairs/sites/maritimeaffairs/files/docs/body/com_2012_494_en.pdf. (access date 10.02.2022).

EC (2018). Commission Communication COM/2018/673. A sustainable bioeconomy for Europe: strengthening the connection between economy, Soc. Environ. https://eur-lex.europa.eu/legal-content/en/ALL/?uri=CELEX%3A52018DC0673. (access date 10.02.2022).

EC (2020a). Commission Communication COM/2020/28. A new circular economy action plan for a cleaner and more competitive Europe. https://eur-lex.europa.eu/legal-content/EN/TXT/?uri=COM%3A2020%3A98%3AFIN.

EC (2020b). Commission Communication COM/2020/381. A farm to fork strategy for a fair, healthy and environmentally-friendly food system. https://eur-lex.europa.eu/legal-content/EN/TXT/?uri=CELEX:52020DC0381.

Enzing, C., Ploeg, M., Barbosa, M., Sijtsma, L., 2014. Microalgae-based products for the food and feed sector: an outlook for Europe. JRC Scientific and policy reports, 19–37.

Enzing, C., et al., European Commission, 2014. Microalgae for food and feed markets, an opportunity for EU's bioeconomy - EU Science Hub - European Commission [Internet]. EU Science Hub. https://ec.europa.eu/jrc/en/news/microalgae-food-and-feed-markets-opportunity-eu-bioeconomy.

Grahl, S., Strack, M., Weinrich, R., Mörlein, D., 2018. Consumer-oriented product development: the conceptualisation of novel food products based on Spirulina (Arthrospira platensis) and resulting consumer expectations. J. Food Qual 2018, 1–11. https://doi.org/10.1155/2018/1919482.

Moons, I., De Pelsmacker, P., Barbarossa, C., 2017. The drivers of the usage intention of Spirulina algae in food in different market segments. Universiteit Antwerpen. Marketing Trends Congr. http://archives.marketing-trends-congress.com/2017/pages/PDF/099.pdf. (access date 20.01.2022).

Moskowitz, H.R., Hartmann, J., 2008. Consumer research: creating a solid base for innovative strategies. Trends Food Sci. Technol. 19 (11), 581–589. https://doi.org/10.1016/j.tifs.2008.01.016.

Pliner, P., Hobden, K., 1992. Development of a scale to measure the trait of food neophobia in humans. Appetite 19 (2), 105–120.

Rahman, K.M., 2020. Food and high value products from microalgae: market opportunities and challenges. Microalgae Biotechnology for Food, Health and High Value Products. Springer, Singapore, pp. 3–27.

Ruiz, J., Olivieri, G., De Vree, J., Bosma, R., Willems, P., Reith, J.H…, Barbosa, M.J., 2016. Towards industrial products from microalgae. Energy Environ. Sci. 9 (10), 3036–3043.

Thomas, Chloé, Symoneaux, Ronan, Pantin-Sohier, Gaelle, Picouet, Pierre, 2020. Isabelle Maître. Perceptions of Spirulina from French Consumers of Organic Products (Matser Thesis. Univertè d'Angers). https://hal.archives-ouvertes.fr/hal-02615769/.

Voort, M.P.J., van der Vulsteke, E., de Visser, C.L.M., 2015. Macroeconomics of algae products. Output report WP2A7.02 of the EnAlgae Project. Swansea. http://www.enalgae.eu/publicdeliverables.htm. (access date 20.01.2022).

Further reading

Colombo, D., 2020. Usbi, la spirulina bio e made in Italy bussa alla Gdo. Freschpointmagazine. https://www.freshpointmagazine.it/retail-marketing/gdo/usbi-spirulina-bio-made-in-italy-gdo/.

CHAPTER 10

Vanity and its impact on nutraceuticals' awareness

Manoel Messias Cavalcante[a], Eduardo de Rezende Francisco[b], Luciana Almeida[a]
[a]ESPM, Sao Paulo, Brazil
[b]FGV EAESP, Sao Paulo, Brazil

10.1 Introduction

The Brazilian population is ageing, and according to Veras (2018), longevity that was once a concern of developed countries has also become a salient issue in developing countries. In Brazil, it reflects progress in several areas, especially in health.

Changes in consumer's lifestyles and advances in medicine have made the 21st century the "Century of Aging" (UNITED NATIONS – United Nations Organisations, 2020). Life expectancy increased from 34.5 to 76.6 years in 1 century, and the population aged 80 years or more will represent 25% of the world's population by 2050. In addition, the population of 65 years or more already exceeds that of 5 years or less in the world. Furthermore, the UN has named the period 2021–2030 the Decade of Healthy Ageing, and will seek to point out, highlight and encourage actions that seek to change the way people think, feel and act in relation to age and ageing, with increased attention to the 17 sustainable development goals (SDGs) in special the third one, to ensure healthy lives and promote well-being for all at all ages (UNDP, 2020; United Nations Brazil, 2021).

Particularly in Brazil, there is a growth in the life expectancy of the elderly, where in 1940, of every thousand people who reached 60 years old, 259 reached 80 years or more. In 2018, of every 1000 seniors aged 65, 637 turned 80. Moreover, Brazilians over 60 years old already exceed 15.7% of the population (32.9 million people). A large part of this population is economically active, concentrates wealth, and is responsible for the income of approximately 25% of Brazilian households. In 2060, the percentage of people over 65 years of age should reach 25.5%, that is, approximately 1 in 4 Brazilians will be elderly (IBGE – Brazilian Institute of Geography and Statistics, 2020a, b; CCdC – With Knowledge Of Cause, 2021).

Case Studies on the Business of Nutraceuticals, Functional and Super Foods
DOI: https://doi.org/10.1016/B978-0-12-821408-4.00009-2
175

In this sense, nutraceuticals emerge as a solution for the elderly consumer who aims to remain healthy and active. Nutraceuticals are described in several studies (Hungenholtz and Smid, 2002; Cândido and Campos, 2005; Kwak and Jukes, 2001; Roberfroid, 2002; Taipina et al., 2002), as foods or part of those that, due to their nutritional characteristics, provide health benefits, in addition to basic nutrition, whether in the prevention or adjuvant treatment. In Brazil, in particular, the term "nutraceutical", first described by DeFelice (1995), over time gained several rereading, currently, nutraceuticals are recognized as dietary supplements.

The Brazilian Health Agency (ANVISA) does not recognize the term nutraceutical, and there is no category of product that uses this definition. The product is considered as a dietary supplement. The ANVISA Resolution No. 243 from July 2018, (RDC No.243) includes products described in other countries as nutraceuticals, but uses the name dietary supplements, although it acknowledges the existence of extensive scientific literature on the subject. According to ANVISA, food supplies are not medicines and therefore do not serve to treat, prevent, or cure diseases. The supplements are intended for healthy people. Its purpose is to provide nutrients, bioactive substances, enzymes, or probiotics in addition to food. The resolution was created in 2018 to ensure the population's access to safe and quality products.

The industry has been offering consumers the most diverse solutions. According to Anunciato (2011), different sectors[a] are now engaged in the creation of new products such as nutricosmetics, nutraceuticals, and cosmeceutics, as shown in Fig. 10.1.

The word "vanity" is often understood, in its everyday interpretation, as something futile, *without content, false appearance or even excess value given to one's own* appearance. Nevertheless, it is also associated with "well-being". This association aimed to give a healthier side for the term "vanity". Previous studies on nutraceuticals, for example, Brower (2005), Boccia and Peluso (2018), Romano (2017), correlated their use with healthy, specially

---

[a]Nutricosmetics are the result of convergence between the cosmetic sand and food industries and are characterized by the ingestion of foods or supplements with the purpose of improving aesthetic aspects (antiwrinkle, antiacne, anticellulite, among others), skin and appendages (Announced, 2011). Cosmeceutical: term introduced by dermatologist Albert Kligman, who defined it as a cosmetic product that exerts therapeutic benefits, but which does not necessarily promote a biological therapeutic activity (Brody, 2005). Nutraceutical: it is defined as any substance that can be considered a food, or part of a food that provides medical or health benefits, including the prevention and treatment of diseases (De Felice, 1995).

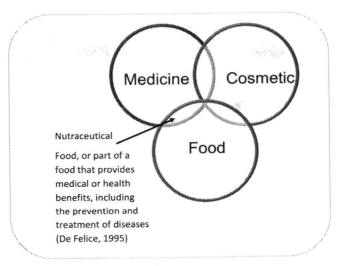

Fig. 10.1 *Solutions developed by the industry.*

addressing the dermatological ageing process, among other research variables, but mostly focused on their efficacy.

Table 10.1 describes the subjects associated with nutraceuticals research in the basis of Google Scholar. It is evident that most studies had addressed the nutraceutical effects on health. However, few of them aimed to relate nutraceuticals to vanity, which indicates a roll of opportunities for studies in this field.

Table 10.1 Search responses —Google scholar.

Search Responses - Google Scholar		
Publication period : 2015 - 2021		

Central Theme	Nutraceutical	
	3,440	

Search Responses for associated themes	Associated Theme	Articles	Percentage
	Health	3,320	26%
	Functional Foods	2,910	23%
	Cosmetics	1,500	12%
	Diabetes	1,810	14%
	Well-being	1,070	8%
	Aging	1,020	8%
	Hypertension	937	7%
	Vanity	31	0.2%

In this sense, Mashorca (2016) pointed out how consumers had become more concerned with improving beauty and self-esteem through the adoption of healthier habits as well the consumption of nutricosmetics aiming to achieve success in social relations.

The central objective of the present chapter consists on presenting a study that sought to evaluate the impact of vanity on the awareness of nutraceutical consumers in Brazil.

The chapter is structured in seven sections, starting the following with a contextualized presentation of the nutraceutical market in Brazil. Section 3 explores the literature on vanity and awareness *to* propose the central hypothesis of the research. Section 4 presents the methodological procedures adopted for conducting field research, as well as for data analysis and interpretation. Section 5 presents the main findings of the research. Sections 6 and 7 seek to demonstrate the real application of study's findings in the Brazilian retail market and propose recommendations to marketing managers in conducting go-to-market strategies and point-of-sales tactics for nutraceuticals sales.

10.2 Nutraceutical market in Brazil

In Brazil, nutraceuticals represent a growing market driven by national particularities. In 2018, Anvisa Resolution (No. 243 of 2018), created the class of dietary supplements which includes nutraceuticals, vitamins, and other dietary supplements. As an example, there was a change in vitamin C's classification. Previously, it was classified as a medicine if it had a dosage above 40 mg—it is currently considered a supplement if it has a dosage up to 500 mg.

The OTC (prescription-free products) market from February/2020 to February/2021 increased around 19%, from U\$ 4.2 billion in 2020 to a total U\$ 4.9 billion.

The OTC market in Brazil consists of more than 150 therapeutic classes. Within this segment, nutraceuticals participate with only six therapeutic classes, accounting approximately for 18% of the total amount. In the same period (February/2020 to February/2021) the nutraceutical market increased from U\$ 690 million to U\$ 922 million, a growth of 31% surpassing the evolution of the total OTC market in the same period (IQVIA PMB report,[b] 2021).

---

[b]IQVIA is a private research institute that audits the Brazilian pharmaceutical market.

Table 10.2 Nutraceuticals' sales performance—Brazilian market.

		Period Feb/20 - Feb/21 (Values in U$ million)		
	Category	**2020**	**2021**	**Evol.**
Nutraceutical Categories	Vitamins	142	254	78%
	Mineral/Calcium	81	97	20%
	Oils (Omega 3 / Cardom)	40	43	8%
	Hairs Vitamin	326	392	20%
	Nutrients	119	142	19%

It is worth to note that the covid-19 pandemic contributed to the Brazilian market growth especially in 2020. The category grew 78% compared to 2019 (IQVIA PMB report, 2021) mostly by the ramp-up on sales of vitamins C and D as consumers followed the nutritionists and physician' recommendations to enhance health. Additionally, Bonfim (2020) related this growth to the consumer's intention to create a body shield for Covid-19's threat of infection and hospitalization.

"The data suggest that nutritional status is a determining factor for a good immune response, and this is achieved in balancing the availability of micro and macronutrients. It is concluded that, at the doses recommended by the current legislation, dietary supplements have a slight impact on the symptoms of COVID-19 disease, when analysed in isolation" (Bonfim, 2020, pp. 10–21).

Bonfim (2020) evaluated vitamins, which had the highest growth as shown in Table 10.3. This growth can be attributed to media efforts in positioning these products to strengthen immunity.

Also, according to Table 10.2, the category of vitamins increased 78% related to 2020. The Brazilian total pharmaceutical market grew 4.1% in 2020 and 10.3% in 2021 (IQVIA PMB report, 2021).

Apart of the Covid19 scenario, Ricardo Ferrari, marketing director of a leader nutraceutical company[c] in Brazil stated: "the sector had already a historical growth ranging from 15 to 20% yearly, (..) the population has adopted new habits and the awareness of vitamins and nutraceuticals aimed at well-being is increasingly in the consumers' routine. Women are continuously aware of the" inside out treatment "concept offered by nutraceuticals".

[c]Interview with the Marketing Director of the company Althaia/Equaliv on 08/03/21 lasting 1 h.

10.3 Literature review

"*Mirror, mirror on the wall, who is the fairest of them all?*". This famous line from the Snow White movie recalls a time in society where princes were the dream of all young women, a time when vanity had not much connection with its current definition. In the story, on one side the young Snow White, in its splendor of beauty and youth, and on the other the Evil Queen, the villain who used witchcraft to remain young and beautiful over the years. In this chapter, the concepts of vanity and awareness are explored from the perspective of prior studies on consumer behaviour and cosmetics products.

10.3.1 Awareness

Awareness is defined as the consumer perception of a product or service regarding the provided information and consumption experience quality (Mowen and Minor, 2003). In this sense, it's recommended to offer as much information as possible aiming to enhance consumer's awareness of a product or service (De Toni et al., 2015).

Guest (1942), entitled "The genesis of brand awareness" inaugurated the literature on brand awareness later endorsed by Keller (1993) and Aaker & Alvarez (2002).

A starting point to create product's awareness consist on understanding why and what a consumer is willing to buy (Sheth et al., 2001). According to Hawkins et al. (2007), customers always seek to base their purchase decisions on two types of fundamentals. The first is based on the attributes presented by the product which includes its communication, packaging, distribution, and even the use of vanity on those marketing strategies to enhance consumer awareness. Secondly, the choice is based on the target audience's vanity.

In this sense, brand knowledge becomes fundamental, as the greater the consumer's knowledge of the product/brand, the greater the possibility of increasing the product/brand purchase intention (Martins et al. 2019). Zubcsek et al. (2017) suggested that customers demonstrate their preferences, and these are opportunities that should be worked out by marketers.

Thus, the consumer's ability to identify and memorize a category, a product, or a brand is what, according to Aaker and Alvarez (2002), constitutes brand awareness. The concept presented reinforces Keller (1993)'s initial proposition that defined brand awareness as the result of two components: remembrance and recognition, which also constitutes, fundamental points for a company's success.

According to Aaker (2002), the brand's influence on the consumer's memory is one of the constituents of brand awareness. In the case of the nutraceutical segment, it is a key element for the recognition by its target audience.

Memory has relevant influence in the "accumulation" of information by customers in relation to the brand, which has a direct influence on the consumer's attitude, called "node force" (Wang and Yang, 2010). Memory will be a definitive element for a consumer to define a brand as unknown or famous (Aaker, 2002).

Keller (2003) acknowledges that the brand knowledge is formed by three factors: (1) functional or symbolic characteristics, arising from the purchase or use, (2) those related to the shopping experience, and (3) brand awareness. The author adds that to evaluate brand awareness it's key to identify the set of variables that influence it, and the consumer behaviour.

It is also relevant to investigate which central benefit offered by the brand is recognized by customers and which variables influence the relationship between the brand and its consumers (Sharifi, 2014).

What desires, needs, or wills link consumers to a brand/category? According to Aaker (1996) brand recognition can be measured through several ways, as for example, the consumer's satisfaction of how the brand meets her/his needs. Having clear which external influences lead the consumer to search for a specific brand can be an interesting start point for building brand awareness.

Driving the customer to experiment a new brand/category is one of the objectives of creating brand awareness. This goal can be performed through marketing mix strategies including pricing, packaging, advertisement, promotion at point of sale as well social networks leads. these efforts might have a significant effect on brand knowledge and purchase intention Sasmita and Suki (2015).

Finally, it is worth highlighting the importance of correct understanding how consumers create and interpret customer awareness once this attitude has a direct effect on perceived quality and consumer decision process to choose a brand (Wu and Ho, 2014; Erdem and Swait, 2004).

10.3.2 Vanity

Throughout human history, people have increased their concern regarding beauty, more than with other valued points in the past (Maffesoli, 1996) and this has a direct effect on people's willingness to spend on beauty products (Goldenberg, 2002).

The concern with self-image has gained more and more relevance in the way that the individual relates to their social groups. This preoccupation emerges from the perspective that a person's success and influence are evaluated by his/her means of conviviality. In this sense, people are consistently investing in beauty and skincare products aiming to associate their self to well-being image (Borelli and Casotti, 2012).

Today, digital media plays a salient role in this context having a great influence on people towards a self-beauty conquest (Santos et al., 2013). Mainstream communication is daily defining and reinforcing vanity patterns for men and women, old and young people.

Self-esteem is highlighted as predictors of people with a greater propensity for new experiences, seen as creative, confident, and sympathetic (Santos et al., 2013). Such personal traits are associated with vanity characteristics Queiroz and Otta (2000), which create beauty patterns focused on achieving the "beautiful body", either using products or even performing aesthetic procedures. According to Strehlau et al. (2015), body self-esteem has a strong connection with vanity, providing a direct relationship in individuals with their self-esteem. Concerns with appearance and its positive impact in relationships and high personal achievements are the factors that compose vanity.

Cosmetics and beauty products promoting appearance-enhancement have strong potential to motivate consumer's awareness by physical vanity. Also, achievements vanity motivates consumer's awareness of items related to status. Both vanities are sources of opportunity for marketing teams to explore these traits in communicating with their consumers (Netemeyer et al., 1995). Regarding consumer's financial conditions to buy beauty products and vanity traits, Mafra et al. (2016) attested that higher the consumer's income greater the expenditure on products and services focused on beauty. In terms of gender, beauty care also has had relevant space in the routine expenses of low-income women (Livramento et al., 2013), reinforcing the relevance of vanity within the female universe.

Women have been empowering themselves in the labour market as well in the society scene. By using cosmetics and well-being products for this purpose, as "allies" for beauty, they seek to achieve success at work and in social relations, a factor driven by society pressure expressed on the "obligation" of women "always to be attractive" Mafra et al. (2016).

On the other hand, awareness of beauty products as an "exclusivity" of the female audiences is changing as the male gender has become vainer in the recent years.

The so-called grooming market—the male cosmetics market in Brazil grew 178.7% in the past decade and yet the country is still in the ninth position in per capita purchases (Euromonitor, 2020) showing the great potential yet to be explored. Sayon et al. (2021) demonstrated that the male cosmetics consumption in Brazil is negatively influenced by income and has a positive influence of vanity and masculinity. Additionally, the grooming market in the country has grown considerably over the years with an increasing variety of solutions for a beautiful body "sculpted" with these products (Sampaio and Ferreira, 2009).

According to the Brazilian Association of the personal hygiene, perfumery, and cosmetics industry (ABIHPEC - Brazilian Association of the Personal Hygiene, Perfumery and Cosmetics Industry 2016), 45% of respondents declared themselves vanity. The data also showed that 54% of the male audience interviewed had frequent habits of going to the beauty salon. This trend confirms what has already been pointed out by Cerqueira et al. (2013) and Sayon et al. (2021). These prior studies stated that the awareness of beauty products was growing among the male audience.

As seen herein, previous literature had investigated the relationship between vanity and awareness for many products such as cosmetics, hair care, skincare, among others, leaving still much room for the study of vanity and nutraceuticals' awareness and consumption.

In this sense, based on the previous literature herein explored, the present research presents the following hypothesis:

H1: Vanity positively impacts consumer nutraceuticals' awareness.

H2: Vanity impacts nutraceuticals' awareness, controlled by gender.

H3: Vanity impacts nutraceuticals' awareness, controlled by age groups.

The next section presents the method adopted to collect data and test the proposed hypothesis.

10.4 Method

For data collection, a *survey* was carried out, whose central objective was to understand whether vanity impacts nutraceuticals' awareness. The research was developed based on the application of a quantitative questionnaire, to seek significant relationships between the constructs addressed in the study (Marconi and Lakatos, 2017). The web tool Survey Monkey was used to collect the participants' responses.

The choice of the survey method is based on the possibility of statistical treatment of the data collected objectively (Leonidou and Katsikeas, 1996).

As the sample size increases, the error range decreases and generates more reliability (Litwin, 1995).

The survey was answered by people living in the Metropolitan Region of Campinas, in the State of São Paulo, and in the Metropolitan Region of São Paulo.[d] The following approach tools were used: WhatsApp, email, Facebook, and by indication and sharing of participants, using the "snow-ball" method, during the months of December 2017–January 2018. To encourage participation in the research, a gift voucher of R$ 100 (equivalent to 16.25 euros or 19.08 dollars in August 2021) was offered as a prize, which was drawn among the respondents.

The questionnaire was composed of four blocks of questions: (1) demographic data of the respondent, (2) self-perception of vanity, (3) knowledge, use, and recommendation of nutraceuticals, and (4) health concern.

The questionnaire presented a nutraceutical definition, by the recommendation of Sheth et al. (2001). The intention was to assess the perception of the product from its precise definition, mitigating different interpretations.

Additionally, seven examples of Brazilian nutraceuticals were presented among the most reference products, being Omega 3, Lycopene, Provitamins, Lutein, Probiotics, and Lactobacilli. The use of examples aimed to facilitate access to consumers' memory regarding the research theme, and, to facilitate the measurement of consumer awareness (Aaker, 2002).

Also, within the questionnaire, the way consumers had access to the products—through the indication of health professionals, friends, or by their own decision, the products were used and recommended, since brand recognition can be measured among other ways through customer satisfaction with the product, which in many cases generates recommendation for acquaintances (Aaker,1996).

Within the questionnaire, awareness was addressed in blocks that evaluated knowledge, perception of health benefit, recommendation, awareness influencers, health care, and pre-existing diseases, seeking to understand the relationship more broadly with the category.

---

[d]Campinas – The Metropolitan Region of Campinas (RMC) has 3.34 million inhabitants, as estimated by IBGE (2021), spread over 20 municipalities in 3791 km². It is the tenth largest metropolitan region in Brazil and the second largest metropolitan region in the State of São Paulo, it is part of the Expanded Metropolitan Complex. São Paulo – The Metropolitan Region of São Paulo (RMSP) is the largest metropolitan region in Brazil, has 22.05 million inhabitants (IBGE, 2021), and one of the ten most populous metropolitan regions in the world, spread over 39 municipalities in 7946.84 km².

To evaluate vanity, the Netemeyer scale was adopted, which had already been used in the relationship between vanity and eating habits by O'Mahony and Hall (2007).

In parallel to the quantitative research work, a passive observation research was conducted in 10 points of sale, seeking to identify the nutraceutical's exhibition and communication considering the real sales scenario in the Brazilian retail context. The use of a mixed-method is recommended once it allows combining the benefits of qualitative and quantitative techniques for data collection and interpretation, expanding the understanding of the studied phenomenon (Creswell, 2014).

The accomplishment of the fieldwork contributed to the development of dialogue with theory, as well as to the elaboration of recommendations for marketing professionals and managers at nutraceuticals industry and retail.

10.4.1 Sample and scale validation

The fieldwork with the quantitative questionnaire in a snowball model obtained a total of 234 respondents and 214 valid answers, concentrated in the Metropolitan Regions of São Paulo and Campinas, presenting an error range of 6.7% and a confidence level of 95%. It was found that 92% of the respondents were over 25 years of age, 59.8% were female, 75.2% had at least a higher level and 54% had an income greater than 6 minimum wages.

The Cronbach's Alpha (1951) was used to verify the reliability of the data. Cronbach's coephycient calculation is a usual method for estimating the confidence and consistency of a given or scale and seeks to evaluate the magnitude in which instrument items are related. Cronbach's alpha has some limitations, but its use is justifiable in assessing the reliability of a scale, recommending it as an acceptable minimum value of 0.6 for each factor as an indicator of acceptable internal consistency (Zambaldi et al., 2014).

For the vanity scale, performed in two groups of questions, Cronbach's alpha found was 0.7445 for the first group (five items) and 0.7700 for the second group (six items). For the scale of knowledge and awareness with seven items, Cronbach's alpha was 0.8420.

10.5 Analysis and results

10.5.1 Sample profile and nutraceutical awareness behaviour

Fig. 10.2 shows the distribution of the data sample and the distribution of nutraceutical awareness by sex. There is no difference in awareness between female and male, as Mann–Whitney test applied (P-value greater than 0.05).

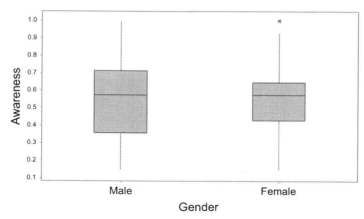

Fig. 10.2 Boxplot: *gender and awareness.*

It is noted that the median awareness is the same for men and women. Fig. 10.2 also shows a more varied awareness for men compared to women.

Table 10.3 shows the balanced distribution of the age group of the data sample and the distribution of nutraceutical awareness by range.

The age group with the highest awareness rates is 45–49 years, in which 25% of people have a propensity equal to or greater than 0.75 (quartile 3). Among the younger ones, between 18 and 34 years old, 25% are prone to at least 0.643, and 50% of them are prone to awareness less than 0.5.

The hypothesis that there is a difference between any of the eight bands when they are compared is not confirmed (P-value of the Kruskal–Wallis Test is 0.108, greater than 0.05).

Table 10.3 Awareness of nutraceuticals by age group.

age group	Respondents	average	Quartile 25%	median	Quartile 75%
18 to 24 years old	17 (7.94%)	0.471	0.286	0.500	0.643
25 to 29 years old	26 (12.15%)	0.511	0.357	0.500	0.643
30 to 34 years old	27 (12.62%)	0.537	0.429	0.571	0.643
35 to 39 years old	34 (15.89%)	0.544	0.357	0.500	0.714
40 to 44 years old	35 (16.36%)	0.578	0.500	0.643	0.714
45 to 49 years old	25 (11.68%)	0.597	0.357	0.643	0.750
50 to 54 years	22 (10.28%)	0.494	0.357	0.500	0.571
55 years or older	28 (13.08%)	0.605	0.500	0.571	0.714
Total	214				

Table 10.4 Recommendation of nutraceuticals.

Recommendation	Respondents	%
I certainly wouldn't recommend	6	2.80%
Probably wouldn't recommend	11	5.14%
Could or could not recommend	55	25.70%
I would probably recommend	85	39.72%
I would certainly recommend	57	26.64%
Total	214	100.00%

In fact, when comparing age groups with 1.8% significance in pairs, it is verified that there is no substantive difference in awareness between the groups.

The questionnaire also collected the willingness to recommend nutraceuticals to those consumers who made use of any of the products mentioned in the survey. According to Table 10.4, the most tend to recommend (66.36% probably or certainly recommend).

10.5.2 Analysis of hypotheses

Hypothesis analysis was performed based on multiple linear regression models. Control variables (gender and age group) were evaluated together, as well as models with interaction. After the segmented analysis, a multivariate regression was performed, considering the main independent variables that could influence the propensity to awareness of nutraceuticals.

10.5.2.1 H1: Vanity impacts nutraceuticals' awareness

Regression considering awareness as a dependent variable and vanity as an independent variable is presented in Table 10.5. The assumptions of regression related to the behaviour of the residuals of the model (normality, independence, and equality of variances of the residues) were validated.

Table 10.5 Hypothesis test H1: vanity × nutraceutical awareness.

Source of variation	d.f.	Quadratic Sum	Quadratic Mean	F Statistics	P-value
regression	1	0.380	0.380	11.15	0.001*
vanity	1	0.380	0.380	11.15	0.001*
error	212	7.220	0.034		
Adjustment test	100	3.695	0.037	1.17	0.204
Pure error	112	3.525	0.031		
Total	213	7.599			

Table 10.5 shows that, with a significance level of 5%, vanity influences awareness. R^2 is 0.050, that is, it is estimated that vanity explains 5% of awareness. It is a low adjustment index, which implies a small power of application in the managerial context, but significant.

The formula resulting from awareness as a function of the vanity is:

Awareness = 0.306 + 0.068*Vanity

The dispersion plot showed that there is a trend of growth in the awareness of nutraceuticals as the vanity scale of the people interviewed increases. The high dispersion of the models corroborates the low value of the coefficient of determination (Appendix A).

10.5.2.2 H2. Vanity impacts nutraceuticals' awareness, controlled by gender

By assuming the independent variables vanity and gender, including testing the hypothesis if they influence awareness together (women with high vanity, for example, have a higher propensity of awareness), the first step verifies the assumptions to apply the regression.

The Anderson–Darling residue normality test resulted in a P-value of 0.599, indicating normality. The residuals also do not show a specific trend when crossed with the adjusted values (equality of variances) or with the order of observations (independence). Therefore, according to the three criteria, the regression is possible. The normality test reached a 5% level of significance, that is, the respondent's gender is not related to awareness, only vanity followed with statistically proven influence (Appendix B).

Table 10.6 shows the regression results. The model adopted explains 6.22% of awareness (R^2), with formula given by:

Awareness = 0.174 + 0.108*Vanity + 0.220*Sex - 0.066*Vanity*Sex

Table 10.6 Hypothesis test H2: vanity × gender × awareness.

Source of variation	d.f.	Quadratic Sum	Quadratic Mean	F Statistics	P-value
regression	3	0.472	0.157	4.64	0.004*
vanity	1	0.385	0.385	11.35	0.001*
Gender	1	0.074	0.074	2.19	0.141
Vanity*Gender	1	0.085	0.085	2.51	0.115
error	210	7.127	0.034		
Adjustment test	131	4.538	0.035	1.06	0.398
Pure error	79	2.589	0.033		
Total	213	7.599			

Table 10.7 Hypothesis test H2: vanity × gender × awareness (no interaction).

Source of variation	d.f.	Quadratic Sum	Quadratic Mean	F Statistics	P-value
regression	2	0.387	0.193637	5.67	0.004
vanity	1	0.385	0.385237	11.27	0.001
Gender	1	0.007	0.007534	0.22	0.639
error	211	7.21	0.034180		
Adjustment test	132	4.62	0.035023	1.07	0.378
Pure error	79	2.59	0.032770		
Total	213	7.5992			

For gender awareness results, the value 1 was assigned for women, and 0 for male:

Female awareness = 0.394 + 0.042*Vanity

Male awareness = 0.174 + 0.108*Vanity

As the regression lines (according to the *different values of the variable dummy* sex) intersect, this shows that women are now more prone to awareness. Therefore, it is not possible to affirm relation between vanity, gender, and awareness (Appendix C).

In addition, Table 10.7 presents the results of the regression of propensity to awareness from the variables vanity and sex — without considering the interaction Vanity*Sex. It is noted that, even without the interaction, the variable Sex is not significant (*P*-value greater than 0.63), reinforcing the conclusion that hypothesis H2 is not supported.

10.5.2.3 H3. Vanity impacts nutraceuticals' awareness, controlled by age groups

To verify the three assumptions to validate the regression with Vanity and Age Group (ranging from 1 to 8) as independent variables, normality tests are presented in Appendix D.

The Anderson–Darling residue normality test had a *P*-value of 0.525, so with a 5% significance level, the residues are normal. The residuals again do not show a specific trend when crossed with the adjusted values (equality of variances) or with the order of observations (independence). Table 10.8 presents the regression results.

With a 5% of significance, again only vanity is related to awareness. The entire model explains 7.67% of the values obtained from nutraceutical awareness. The regression formula follows below:

Awareness = 0.280 + 0.057*Vanity + 0.004*Age group + 0.003*Vanity*Age group

Table 10.8 Hypothesis test H3: vanity × age group × awareness.

Source of variation	d.f.	Quadratic Sum	Quadratic Mean	F Statistics	P-value
regression	3	0.582	0.194	5.8	0.001*
vanity	1	0.036	0.036	1.08	0.301
age group	1	0.000	0.000	0.01	0.915
Vanity*Age group	1	0.003	0.003	0.09	0.765
	21				
error	0	7.017	0.033		
	18				
Adjustment test	3	6.359	0.035	1.43	0.138
Pure error	27	0.658	0.024		
	21				
Total	3	7.599			

You cannot graph the formula linearly when you have more than one independent variable in the equation.

When testing whether only the age group influences the propensity to awareness, the regression is valid to be applied. Appendix E presents the residual graphs of the model (normality tests for age and awareness).

The normality of the residues was confirmed by the Anderson–Darling test, which presented a P-value of 0.418. The independence of the residues and the equality of variances were confirmed by the absence of a pattern in the graphs on the right.

Table 10.9 presents the regression model between age group and awareness.

The age group is significant in the 5% model because the P-value is less than 0.05. R^2 indicates that age explains 2.07% of propensity to awareness, and the positive coefficient estimates that the higher the awareness, the older the age group:

Awareness = 0.489 + 0.013*Age group

Table 10.9 Hypothesis test H3: age-to-E-awareness ratio.

Source of variation	d.f.	Quadratic Sum	Quadratic Mean	F Statistics	P-value
regression	1	0.158	0.157	4.49	0.035 *
age group	1	0.158	0.157	4.49	0.035 *
error	212	7.442	0.035		
Adjustment test	6	0.230	0.038	1.09	0.367
Pure error	206	7.212	0.035		
Total	213	7.599			

Table 10.10 H3 hypothesis test: vanity ratio and age group (no interaction). Summary of hypothesis results.

hypothesis	Supported	observation
H1: Vanity positively impacts consumer awareness of nutraceuticals	Yes	The P-value of the F-test of the regression of propensity to Consumption from Vanity is significant (0.001). Nevertheless, the power of explanation (R^2) is low (0.050).
H2: Vanity has an impact on the nutraceuticals consumption with variations according to gender	No	The variables Sex and Vanity*Sex were non-significant (P-value greater than 0.11) in the model together with Vanity to explain the propensity to Consumption, to a significance level (α) of 5%. Similarly, the variable Sex was non-significant (P-value greater than 0.63) even without the interaction with Vanity.
H3: Vanity has an impact on the consumption of nutraceuticals with variations according to age	Partially Supported	The variables Age (Age Group) and Vanity*Age were non-significant (P-value greater than 0.76)in the model together with Vanity to explain the propensity to Consumption. Notifiedly, the variable Age was significant (P-value of 0.015) in the model in conjunction with Vanity (P-value less than 0.001), without the interaction with Vanity.

The propensity to awareness increased 1.3% for each unit over the age group. The age group influences the increase of awareness.

In the Kruskal–Wallis test, with the level of 5% there is no difference in awareness between age groups if they are compared in pairs. This is because the variability of age groups is similar. In addition, the means and the medians are close, as shown in Appendix F.

The dispersion between the awareness data according to the eight age groups is not very illustrative because the idea of the scatter plot is to deal with continuous data, and the age group is qualitative ordinal and class limits are integer values.

Table 10.10 presents the results of the regression model of awareness from Vanity and Age Group, without considering the interaction.

After analysing Vanity and Age Group in isolation without the interaction between both, a P-value was lower than 0.05, which suggests that awareness increases as Vanity and Age Group increase.

Awareness = 0.2263 + 0.0722 Vanity + 0.01428 Age Group

There is no multilinearity between Vanity and Age Group, according to the variance inflation factor indicator calculated in the model. The model presented in Table 10.9 shows R^2 of 7.62% (Appendix G).

After the validation and understanding of the response analysis tool originated by the 214 questionnaires, the following response to the impact of vanity on the awareness of the nutraceutical consumer, described in Table 10.10, with the results of the P-value and R^2.

With the confirmation of the impact of vanity on the awareness of nutraceutical consumers, the next section seeks to analyse how the category has used this factor in its work at the point of sale.

10.5.3 Points-of-sale (POS) observational research: Results and analysis

In contrast to the survey findings, the observational research evidenced that most nutraceuticals manufacturers, mostly pharmacy industries, are adopting a conservative communication strategy to gather consumer's attention focusing their arguments in medical recommendations instead of vanity-related factors, well-being, and self-esteem.

Fig. 10.3 demonstrates a planogram at a Brazilian drugstore. It is evident that there is a bare effort to associate nutraceuticals with well-being,

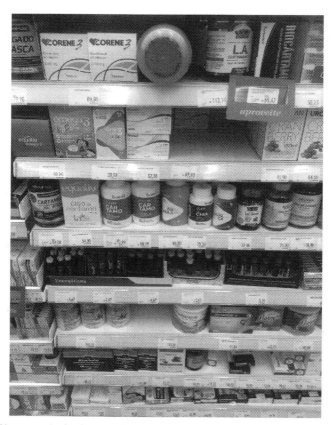

Fig. 10.3 *Nutraceuticals planogram at POS (POS-1).*

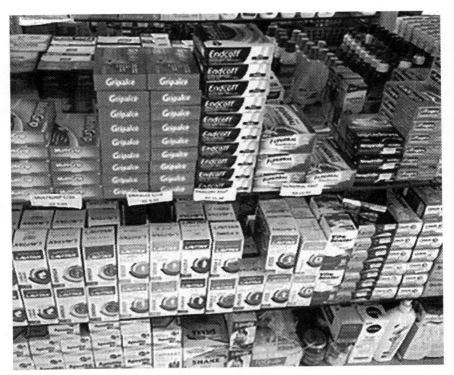

Fig. 10.4 *Nutraceuticals planogram at POS (POS-2).*

self-esteem, or even images related to vanity. The planogram portrays a sale and communication strategy largely used to promote OTC medicines. Fig. 10.4 shows nutraceutical products in the same shelf of the medicines for pain.

According to Table 10.2, vitamins are the second market for nutraceuticals in Brazil. However, their communication at the point-of-sale remains conservative and distant from the arguments evidenced in the survey findings, associating brand awareness with vanity.

Besides the planogram, packaging and communication are mostly based on medical evidence instead of solutions for a healthier life. Another strategy that reflects the adoption of OTC strategies for nutraceuticals communication consists of the use of bundle sales and promotions like 3 for 2 prices (Fig. 10.5).

Some companies begin to change the communication enhancing packaging design towards a well-being approach. However, the marketing action at the POS still faces salient challenges, as shown in Fig. 10.6.

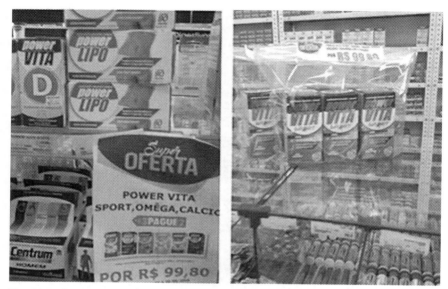

Fig. 10.5 *Current nutraceutical's promotion tactics (POS-3).*

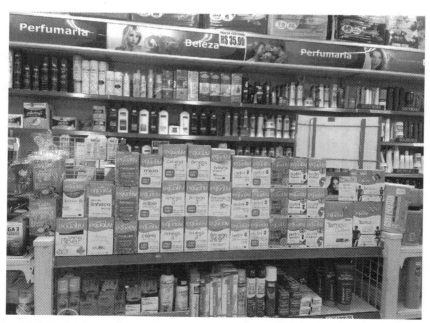

Fig. 10.6 *Packaging redesign and planogram tactics (POS-4).*

Additionally, websites from the four Brazilian major brands in the segment of nutraceuticals, demonstrated two positionings: medicine approach and well-being approach.

10.6 Conclusion

Ageing is a present issue among developed and emergent economies' key concerns. The theme is also addressed by ONU's SDGs through the third goal demonstrating an urgent call for action to ensure health and well-being for all. Additionality, there are a growing number of academic studies addressing the theme of healthy ageing. Yet, studies on consumer behaviour regarding nutraceuticals offers a vast room for investigation.

The present chapter explored the nutraceuticals market in Brazil and its rapidly growth evidenced by the consumer awareness and consumption. Moreover, the findings demonstrated the positive relation between nutraceuticals' awareness and vanity, as evidence that consumers associate this category not as medicine but as salient contributor for their well-being and body appearance. Age was found to have a significant moderation in the relationship between vanity and awareness.

The findings also pointed out the manufactures myopia to explore planograms, packaging, and promotions at POS. These results evidenced an opportunity for marketers to employ a new approach to promote consumer awareness focusing on well-being and vanity elements rather than the one mostly employed by the current players focused on medicine benefits.

10.7 Management recommendations

Based on the main research evidence, some recommendations are offered above:

1. Concerning the "Universal Sales Proposition", packaging might explore more aspects of vanity.

Efforts in communication, packaging, and other points of contact with the consumer should be linked with a universal sales proposition that enhances well-being benefits associated with beauty care.

In partnership with a Brazilian manufacture of nutraceuticals, this recommendation was adopted in the relaunch of nutraceutical products as shown in Fig. 10.7. The company's packaging strategy presents a disruptive model regarding the current category's approach. Consumer awareness was stimulated by the images representing people that appear well-being and

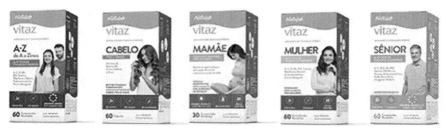

Fig. 10.7 *Relaunch with changes in packaging design.*

body care as elements linked with vanity. Also, the image aimed to create recognition and empathy for each public.

2. Communication of the nutraceutical's benefits according to the age group.

The findings demonstrated that as the age group increases, the awareness of the consumer of nutraceuticals evolves. Based on this reasoning, a proper product positioning for each age group should be an opportunity for market expansion.

Appendix

Appendix A: Awareness dispersion graph versus vanity—hypothesis 1

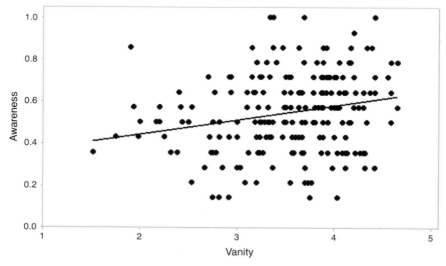

Appendix B: Normality test—gender

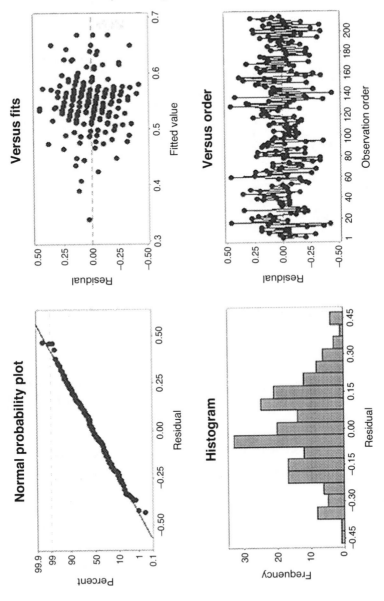

Appendix C: Dispersion plot of the relationship awareness versus vanity and gender

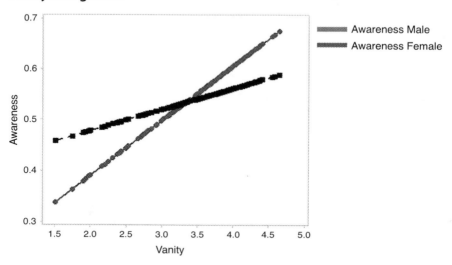

Appendix D: Normality test—age group

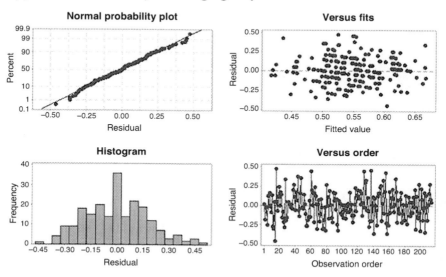

Appendix E: Normality test—age and awareness

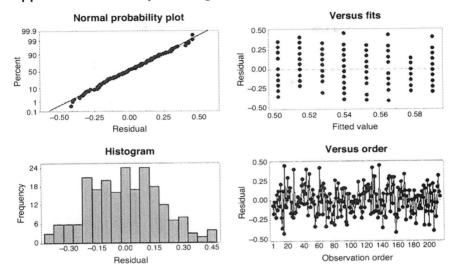

Appendix F: Variability of age groups and dispersion plot by age group

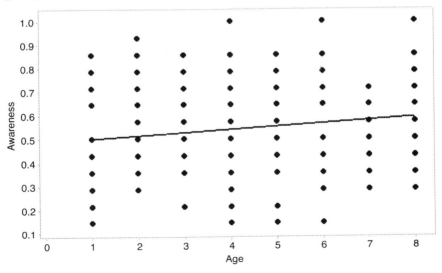

Appendix G: Normality test—vanity and age group

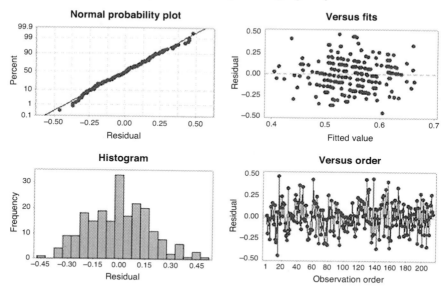

References

Aaker, D., 2002. Building Strong Brands London. *Simon & Shuster.*

Aaker, D.A., Alvarez del Blanco, R.M.P., 2002. Construir marcas poderosas. Gestión 2000.

Aaker, D.A., 1996. Measuring brand equity across products and markets. Calif. Manage. Rev. 38 (3), 106–120.

ABIHPEC - Brazilian Association of the Personal Hygiene, Perfumery and Cosmetics Industry. (2016). 54% of them regularly attend beauty salons and barbershops without the slightest fear. https://abihpec.org.br/release/mercado-masculino-de-hppc-segue-em-crescimento/ (Accessed April 20, 2021).

Anunciato, T.P. (2011). Nutricosméticos Doctoral dissertation, University of São Paulo.

Boccia, F., Peluso, F., 2018. Future food and economic sustainability: the nutraceutical technology. Quality-Access to Success 19 (167).

Bomfim, J.H.G.G., da Silveira Gonçalves, J., 2020. Dietary supplements, immunity and COVID-19: what is the evidence? VITTALLE-Journal of Health Sciences 32 (1), 10–21.

Borelli, F.C., Casotti, l.M, 2012. How to be a man and be beautiful? An exploratory study on the relationship between masculinity and beauty awareness. Electronic Administration Read 18 (2), 400–432.

Brower, V., 2005. A nutraceutical a day may keep the doctor away: consumers are turning increasingly to food supplements to improve well-being when pharmaceuticals fail. EMBO Rep. 6 (8), 708–711.

Candido, l.M.B., Campos, a.M., 2005. Functional foods. A review. Bulletin of the sbcta 29 (2), 193–203.

CCdC - With Knowledge Of Cause (2021). Platform Longeviver. https://longeviver.com/ (accessed May 12, 2020).

Cerqueira, A.C., de Oliveira, R.C.R., Honório, J.B., Bergamo, F.V.M., 2013. Cosmetic consumer behavior: an exploratory study. Magazine trainers 6 (1), 128.

Creswell, J.W., 2014. Research Design. Qualitative, Quantitative, and Mixed Methods Approaches (4th edition). Thousand Oaks, CA Sage Publications.

De Felice, Sl., 1995. The nutraceutical revolution: its impact on food industry R&D. Trends Food Sci. Technol. 6 (2), 59–61.

De Toni, D., Fill, R.A, Larentis, F., Milan, G.S, 2015. Influence of image and perception of value on the intention to purchase chicken meat: a quantitative study. Race 14 (3), 1005–1034.

Erdem, T., Swait, J., 2004. Brand credibility, brand consideration and choice. Journal of consumer research 31 (1), 191–198 v.n.

Euromonitor (2020), "Beauty and personal care industry reports", www.portal.euromonitor. com/portal (accessed May 18, 2020).

Goldenberg, M., 2002. Naked & Dressed: Ten Anthropologists Reveal the Culture of Rio's Body. Record Publishing House, Rio de Janeiro, p. 414.

Guest, L.P., 1942. The genesis of brand awareness. J. Appl. Psychol. 26 (6), 800.

Hawkins Del I, M.D.L., Best Roger, J., 2007. Consumer Behavior: Building Marketing Strategy. McGraw-Hill/Irwin, California.

Hugenholtz, J., Smid, E.J., 2002. Nutraceutical production with food-grade microorganisms. Curr. Opin. Biotechnol. 13 (5), 497–507.

IBGE - Brazilian Institute of Geography and Statistics (2021). Estimativas da população residente nos Municípios brasileiros com data de referência em 1° de julho de 2021. https://ftp.ibge.gov.br/Estimativas_de_Populacao/Estimativas_2021/ (accessed August 12, 2021).

IBGE - Brazilian Institute of Geography and Statistics (2020a). In 2018, life expectancy was 76.3 years. https://agenciadenoticias.ibge.gov.br/agencia-sala-de-imprensa/2013-agencia-de-noticias/releases/26104-em-2018-expectativa-de-vida-era-de-76-3-anos (accessed May 12, 2020).

IBGE - Brazilian Institute of Geography and Statistics (2020b). PNAD-Covid19. IBGE supporting the fight against COVID-19. https://covid19.ibge.gov.br/pnad-covid/.

Keller, k.L., 1993. Conceptualizing, measuring, and managing customer-based brand equity. Journal of Marketing 57 (1), 1–22.

Keller, K.L., 2003. Brand synthesis: the multidimensionality of brand knowledge. Journal of consumer research 29 (4), 595–600.

Kwak, N.S., Jukes, D.J., 2001. Functional foods. Part 1: the development of a regulatory concept. Food Control 12 (2), 99–107.

Leonidou, L.C., Katsikeas, C.S., 1996. The export development process: an integrative review of empirical models. Journal of international business studies 27 (3), 517–551.

Litwin, M.S., Fink, A., 1995. How to Measure Survey Reliability and Validity (vol. 7). Thousand Oaks, CA Sage Publications.

Livramento, M.N., Hor-Meyll, L.F., Pessôa, L.A.G.D.P., 2013. Valores que motivam mulheres de baixa renda a comprar produtos de beleza. RAM. Revista de Administração Mackenzie 14, 44–74.

Maffesoli, M., 1996. The Contemplation of the World: Figures of Community Style. University of Minnesota Press, Minnesota.

Mafra, A.L., Castro, F.N., de Araújo Lopes, F., 2016. Investment in beauty, exercise, and self-esteem: Are they related to self-perception as a romantic partner? Evolutionary Psychological Science 2 (1), 24–31.

Marconi, M.D.A., Lakatos, E.M., 2017. Research Techniques: Planning and Execution of Research, Sampling and Research Techniques, Preparation, Analysis and Interpretation of Data. Fundamentos de metodologia científica. Atlas. GEN., São Paulo, SP, p. 277.

Martins, J., Costa, C., Oliveira, T., Gonçalves, R., Branco, F., 2019. How smartphone advertising influences consumers' purchase intention. Journal of Business Research 94, 378–387.

Mashorca, K.S., Spers, E.E., by Proença Vetucci, J., Silva, Da, H.M., R., 2016. Beauty and vanity in relation to new types of food: a study on the market of nutricosmetics. Revista Brasileira de Marketing 15 (3), 401–417.

Mowen, J.C., Minor, M.S., 2003. Consumer behavior. Prentice Hall, São Paulo.

Netemeyer, R.G., Burton, S., Lichtenstein, D.R., 1995. Trait aspects of vanity: measurement and relevance to consumer behavior. Journal of Consumer Research 21 (4), 612–626.

O'Mahony, B., Hall, J., 2007. An exploratory analysis of the factors that influence food choice among young women. International Journal of Hospitality & Tourism Administration 8 (2), 51–72.

Queiroz, R.D.S., Otta, E., 2000. Beauty in focus: cultural and psychobiological constraints in the definition of body aesthetics. The Body of the Brazilian: Studies of Aesthetics and Beauty. SENAC, São Paulo, pp. 13–66.

Roberfroid, M., 2002. Functional food concept and its application to prebiotics. Dig. Liver Dis. 34, S105–S110.

Romano, M.C., 2017. The role of nutrition and Nutraceutical for the well-being of skin. European Journal of Aesthetic Medicine & Dermatology 7.

Sampaio, R., Ferreira, R.F., 2009. Beauty, identity and market. Psicologia em Revista 15 (1), 120–140.

Santos, A.R.M.D., Silva, E.A.P.C.D., Moura, P.V.D., Dabbico, P., Silva, P.P.C.D., Freitas, C.M.S.M.D., 2013. A busca pela beleza corporal na feminilidade e masculinidade. Rev. bras. ciênc. mov, 135–142.

Sasmita, J., Suki, N.M., 2015. Young consumers' insights on brand equity: effects of brand association, brand loyalty, brand awareness, and brand image. International Journal of Retail & Distribution Management 43 (3), 276–292.

Sayon, M., de Almeida, L.F., Ponchio, M.C., 2021. It's time for men to groom up!. Journal of Consumer Marketing 38 (2), 147–158.

Sheth, J., Mittal, B., Newman, B., 2001. Customer behavior: Going beyond consumer behavior. Atlas, São Paulo.

Sharifi, S.S., Esfidani, M.R., 2014. The impacts of relationship marketing on cognitive dissonance, satisfaction, and loyalty: The mediating role of trust and cognitive dissonance. International Journal of Retail & Distribution Management 42 (6), 553–575.

Strehlau, V.I., Claro, D.P., Laban, S.A., 2015. Does vanity drive the awareness of cosmetics and surgical aesthetic procedures in women? An exploratory investigation. Revista de Administração (São Paulo) 50, 73–88.

Taipina, M.S., Fontes, M.A.D.S., Cohen, V.H., 2002. Alimentos funcionais-nutracêuticos. Hig. aliment 16 (100), 28–29.

UNDP (2020). Sustainable development goals. https://www.br.undp.org/content/brazil/pt/home/sustainable-development-goals.html (accessed August 12, 2021).

UNITED NATIONS - United Nations Organisations (2020). UN Summit discusses population aging and sustainable development. https://nacoesunidas.org/cupula-da-onu-discute-envelhecimento-populacional-e-desenvolvimento-sustentavel/ (accessed May 12, 2020).

United Nations Brazil (2021). About our work to achieve the sustainable development goals in Brazil. 2021. https://brasil.un.org/pt-br/sdgs (accessed August 12, 2021).

Veras, R.P., Oliveira, M., 2018. Aging in Brazil: the construction of a model of care. Science & Public Health 23, 1929–1936.

Wang, X., Yang, Z., 2010. The effect of brand credibility on consumers' brand purchase intention in emerging economies: The moderating role of brand awareness and brand image. Journal of global marketing 23 (3), 177–188.

Wu, S.I., Ho, L.P., 2014. The influence of perceived innovation and brand awareness on purchase intention of innovation product—an example of iPhone. International Journal of Innovation and Technology Management 11 (04), 1450026.

Zambaldi, F., Da Costa, F.J., Ponchio, M.C., 2014. Mensuração em marketing: Estado atual, recomendações e desafios. Revista Brasileira de Marketing 13 (2), 1–27.

Zubcsek, P.P., Katona, Z., Sarvary, M., 2017. Predicting mobile advertising response using consumer colocation networks. Journal of Marketing 81 (4), 109–126.

Conclusions

The nutraceutical and superfood industry is an excellent example of the turbulence that we are experiencing in these times. The advent of sustainability awareness, the emergence of healthy lifestyles, and pandemic events characterise this decade. Consumers have access to a broad range of information and perceive the importance of changing their food approach: people seek foods that associate benefits with consumption. This book shows that a culture that nudges healthy eating is emerging.

The vast interest in nutraceuticals and superfoods has intensified new product development. Companies operating in the food, pharmaceutical, or cosmeceutical industries have launched new products on the market with the intent of meeting emerging needs and market demand.

The size of the global market for nutraceuticals and superfoods has registered a progressive growth in the last 10 years. As it emerges from the book, the blurring of industries and the convergence between food, pharma, and cosmeceutical sectors has reshaped competitive dynamics among players. Therefore, firms need to define their competitive positioning and advantage adequately. In the above-described scenario, the investigation of consumers becomes of primary importance. This book shows methods, techniques, and applications of consumer science and research, and it underlines how important it is to integrate a multidisciplinary approach—like the combination of consumer science and strategic marketing—when planning the development of a new product or, more in general when designing, a strategy.

The selected cases outline some issues that characterise strategies for nutraceutical products that ranging from ethical motives to communication issues.

A key thematic is implementing nutraceutical features to achieve successful product differentiation.

We know that nutraceutical components play a crucial role in achieving differentiation. The presence of nutraceuticals can facilitate the launching of new products that can target different needs: we have seen that the growing consumers' awareness of healthy properties of foods can create facilitating conditions for successful new products launches.

Therefore, it is pivotal to have a detailed knowledge of the market and maintain a market orientation to avoid market failures.

A key element is the relationship between product features and differentiation.

The diffusion of nutraceutical products has opened new market possibilities for companies operating in various industries. In a business that is booming, where new products are launched to meet emerging needs and reach new customers, it becomes hard to pursue differentiation in the long run. The degree of competition has increased in the industry: small industries with favourable growth rates and profitability often become global industries. Margins and profits attract competitors, and as the number of competitors grows, there is a proliferation of new products.

Then, it becomes pivotal to understand consumers. New competitive trajectories emerge, and it is interesting to highlight how some companies combine consolidated or traditional issues in product marketing with recent developments (such as nutraceutical components).

The book underlines how mixing nutraceutical features and other product characteristics can create a competitive advantage. New nutraceutical trends could emerge, such as "made in" nutraceuticals: combining the country of origin with product features can help achieve a differentiation based on traditional competitive leverage, such as location and country of origin. The discussion that emerges in the book about the efficacy of linking nutraceutical features to a "made in" concept or to traditional local food opens to a debate on a new market niche in this promising industry. Furthermore, the growing competition has opened a debate in some specific categories of nutraceuticals: companies are focusing on analysing value and margins to improve a firm's competitiveness.

The book also introduces the role that nutraceuticals can have in developing solutions for ensuring access to nutrients to specific populations. It underlined the ethical aspect of this industry.

As we can see, nutraceuticals and superfoods are changing. It emerges a differentiation of products designed according to specific strategic purposes, ethical issues, and market orientation.

The need to adopt a multidisciplinary approach emerges from this reading: integrating multiple perspectives capable of listening to consumers' voices will help companies operating in this business.

As we have seen, it is impossible to gain precise information about market trends and size, even because this business lacks regulation and is highly dynamic. This book provides suggestions about how the industry will evolve. It shows how players will compete in the future: this is possible because we have included in the reading emerging insights from research, examples of field research and cases of companies.

In our view, this publication's main lesson is that we need multidisciplinarity inside companies' management and research and when talking to professionals.

Index

Page numbers followed by "*f*" and "*t*" indicate, figures and tables respectively.

Printed in the United States
by Baker & Taylor Publisher Services